By The Same Author

2010: *Lose Weight Now!*

2003: *The Psychodynamics of the Unconscious.* Intapsy
Publications, London.

2002: *Mind Castles.* Intapsy Publications, London.

STOP SMOKING NOW!

A Practical Mind Technique to Stop Smoking Completely, Easily and Effectively

Antony Maurice-Nneke

Eloquent Books

First Published in 2010

British Library Cataloguing in Publication Data

A catalogue reference for this book is available from the British Library

ISBN: 978-1-60911-837-2

Published by Eloquent Books
An Imprint of Strategic Book Group
P O BOX 333, Durham CT 06422, USA.
www.strategicbookgroup.com

TO MY FAMILY

I love you all. I am always inspired and uplifted by your care and attention. I thank you all for giving me the strength and energy with which to carry on.

Acknowledgment

I am immensely grateful to my daughter Laetitia who brings me joy from day to day. I am grateful to her for her great support during the period of my mother's long illness and her subsequent death. At times during this sad period it felt like I was the child and Laetitia was the parent, her caring skills were so much accomplished for someone of her young age. It is moments like this that beg the question about whether grief is an illness!

My work on this book suffered during this sad period but Laetitia encouraged me to complete the book and she arranged and promoted some of my public workshops on the topic of this book. My subtitle for this book says exactly what the book is about but it was Laetitia who suggested the main title of the book, **Stop Smoking Now!,** which I have now adopted as a series title and used for my book *Lose Weight Now!*.

I give thanks to Laetitia for her great words of wisdom, comfort and for the way she helped me to get over my deep feeling of sadness, hollowness and emptiness that followed the wake of the sad loss of my mother.

I am very grateful to Angelina and Emmanuel for helping to look after my mother and I thank other members of my family for being present at the funeral. I thank everyone for being there for me with huge support. I love you all.

Contents

Introduction

It is all in the state of mind, success in anything you do begins in the mind.

THE BASIC IDEA OF THE MIND TECHNIQUE IN THIS BOOK

This book is a practical application of some of the ideas and fundamental principles of mind power technique that I introduced in my book, *Mind Castles* (2002) and applied in my book *Lose Weight Now!* The book reveals the secret power of the mind and gives the individual the power to achieve success by making use of those secrets. The book presents a novel approach to stop smoking which is simple, fun to practise and highly effective. It demonstrates a unique practical mind technique that enables the individual to give up smoking easily, completely, effectively and effortlessly.

The book contains some of the essential secret weapons which an individual needs in order to look good and feel good in every way and regain the energy and stamina that he or she has lost by the ravages of tar and nicotine from inhaling tobacco smoke into the lungs in smoking cigarettes, cigars or pipe. The book teaches a special method of relaxation that enables the individual wishing to give up smoking to accomplish his or her objectives quickly and effectively.

In practising the special method of deep relaxation that the book teaches, some people may feel light and weightless when they relax. They may feel as light as if they can just float away. It is usual to feel this way but it is not a necessary part of the application of this method. What is necessary is that the individual must feel relaxed

However, if an individual can feel light during the moment of deep relaxation, he or she is beginning to acquire the feeling of being in control. This is the feeling which this book creates for individuals as they inculcate the habit of relaxation in the special way that is taught in this book.

When an individual has this feeling of being in control constantly in his or her mind, he or she will know that he or she is beginning to accomplish the goal of giving up smoking for success begins in the mind. The next stage is for the individual to translate the feeling into the physical activities that will make the feeling become his or her reality so that he or she can experience the real action of giving up smoking and do so easily and effortlessly. The simple mind techniques in this book are intended to enable any individual to harness the power to bring about the changes which he or she requires in life, be it in giving up smoking or in any other venture where the goal of the individual is to achieve success.

This book shows the way to achieve success in giving up smoking and it shows, truly, the way to achieve success in any goal or anything you do; how to be what you want to be, how to do things seriously in a positive way so that you do them successfully. It shows how to erect a solid foundation to the mind castles which people build from day to day.

The strong message in the book is that you will get what you want for what you want is what you get. This means that when you have a positive mental attitude and your mind is fully focused on what you want, the goals which you aspire to attain become easily attainable by you. Any person who desires to give up smoking would be successful in giving up smoking easily and effectively if the person has a positive mental attitude and a strong belief in his or her own ability to attain the desired objective of giving up smoking easily and effectively.

The success comes through an intentional positive action. Any person who can talk the talk about giving up smoking must walk the walk to realize the goal by putting the talk into action. This book is about responsible positive action which brings about positive changes by helping the individual to give up smoking easily and effectively.

This book shows you how to inculcate a positive mental attitude, how to acquire self belief, self esteem and how to project a positive self image in whatever you do. The book takes you through the actions that you must perform, and the attitudes that you must adopt in order to achieve success in giving up smoking.

If you can bring yourself to believe that you have the power within you to bring to reality anything that you can conceive as possible in your life, then you will be truly on your way to achieving your desired objective of giving up smoking and you will do so easily and effortlessly. The conception of the possibility of the idea, and the reality of it, begin with effective thought bricks which form the foundation of your own mind castle in relation to giving up smoking easily and effortlessly. This idea will become much clearer to you in chapter one when we consider the fundamental principles of the mind technique that I introduce in this book.

The claim of this book is that every individual has the power within him or her to achieve the goals and objectives that he or she wishes to achieve in life, to make whatever changes he or she wishes to make in his or her life successfully. In order to do this seriously and conscientiously, the individual has to, first, acknowledge the enormous power within him or her and, secondly, make use of that power by doing something new or, at least, doing something different from what he or she has been doing in the past.

The emphasis here, as in 'walk the walk', mentioned above, is in positive action which consists in the practise of the relaxation exercises in this book, doing something new in order to accomplish one's goals and aspirations.

A person's acknowledgement and utilization of his or her inner power for success entails the belief that there is no limit to what he or she can accomplish, legitimately, with his or her mind except the limitations which he or she, wilfully, imposes on himself or herself by distorted thoughts and self doubt. The power of the mind is utilized in thought processes and this is manifested by an individual's actions in so far as thoughts precede actions.

By following all the positive ideas in this book and the actions that they invoke, the serious reader will develop a positive attitude towards the desired goal of giving up smoking. This will help him or her to give up smoking easily and effectively.

The reader will also develop a great confidence in his or her ability to succeed in any chosen venture and he or she will be ready, willing, and able to embark on the road to success. The essential ingredients that are required for a recipe for success in giving up smoking by the method of deep relaxation and mental programming are in this book.

The effective use of these essential ingredients will propel any serious reader to the road of success in giving up smoking easily and effortlessly when he or she has read the book attentively from the beginning to the end and practised the techniques as advised.

A person's decision to read this book brings that person a step nearer to that road; and he or she will be walking firmly on that road with the head held high by the time he or she has read to the end of this book when he or she has read the book with concentrated attention supported by a clear understanding and performance of the necessary actions which an individual must take to achieve the success that he or she desires. Some of these actions consist in practising all the relaxation exercises for giving up smoking which are given in this book.

There is a clear user-friendly advantage to this book which is in the way that things look familiar to the reader as he or she reads through the pages of the book. This is partly because of the simplicity of the ideas, the relaxation exercises and the way in which the ideas have been presented in this book and partly because our subject matter, *Giving up smoking*, is a subject which is of great public interest. Many people have an interest to give up smoking but they fob themselves off the attempt to give up smoking with pathetic excuses.

This book provokes you into positive action. It urges you to avoid the temptation of using pathetic excuses to hold on to an unwanted, unhealthy and dangerous habit. It urges you to do something as a positive concern for your health, to practise the simple techniques discussed in the book because simple techniques always work. They work because they are simple.

In my work as psychotherapist, lecturer, counsellor and life coach in London I organize regular seminars and workshops on mind power techniques such as techniques for *Memory (MRT)* as developed in *Mind Castles* (2002) and applied in *Lose Weight Now!*, workshops on losing weight, giving up smoking and others. These workshops are held regularly at various venues in London. I have also worked in the area of sports translating the principles of depth psychology into the practical areas of sports performance.

In this respect, I have used some of the simple mind power techniques discussed in this book to help my clients, many sports people, athletes, boxers, footballers, gymnasts, and tennis players, to lose weight, stop smoking and to gain a great confidence in themselves. My work with these sports people has enabled them to achieve success in their own sports by attaining a much desired personal best (PB) performance in their sports.

As a result of all these, I have every confidence in anyone reading this book for the serious purpose of giving up smoking. If this is your intention for reading this book, you must spend time to try out all the positive suggestions given and participate fully in the deep relaxation exercises given in *the practice sessions* in the book.

THE PRACTICE SESSIONS

This is a practical book for giving up smoking. As I mentioned above, if a person is able to talk the talk about giving up smoking, then that person must be prepared to put the talk into practical action and walk the walk which will lead him or her to the fulfilment of the desired goal. The *practice sessions* are an essential part of the positive action in this book and they are intended to help the serious reader to develop a relaxed attitude in mind and body. This will help him or her to focus the mind sharply on the desired objective of giving up smoking.

The *Key Points to Remember* which are given in the various sections of this book are a quick reference to the issues raised in a particular discussion and provides a brief summary of the key points in the discussion. The act of remembering these key points forms part of the practical action in this book for one has to remember the ideas in order to put them into practice.

This book is in itself an exploration into the powers of the human mind. Our underlying thesis is that success in anything we do begins in the mind. *It is all in the mind.* This becomes obvious as one reads through the pages of this book. As I mentioned above, if you are reading this book with a serious intention to give up smoking, you must practise the simple techniques in the book because simple techniques work. They work because they are simple. The simple techniques in this book are part of the simple techniques that I use every week in my own work and in the workshops that I organize.

In addition to helping readers to learn how to stop smoking completely, easily and effectively, the readers will also learn the following from reading the book.

- The secrets of how the human mind works.
- How to use effective thought bricks to erect an impregnable mind castle.
- How to relax and take control of any situation.
- How to recognise the effects of stress and anxiety in personal life.
- How to acquire confidence, self esteem and self worth.
- How to formulate goals and make plans for the future.
- How to make a plan of action to achieve a specific goal.
- How to visualise for success in any venture.

You can also view this book as an introduction to psychocybernetics, the application of solid thought bricks as a foundation for the construction of mind castles in making radical changes in life. In this respect, the book is a journey into a new world, a new way of doing things, a new method of approach to personal and social problems, a quest for self development.

We begin the journey or quest in the next section with a preparatory exercise to set the psychical system in motion so that you will feel relaxed. When you perform this exercise properly, diligently, you will notice that you will feel relaxed in mind and body from that moment onwards.

CHAPTER ONE
Essential Preliminary Steps to Stop Smoking

When you visualize something, you can make it a material reality. If you are able to visualize yourself as a non-smoker and think constantly that you are a non-smoker, then this will certainly become your reality. This is the essence of visualization: whatever you visualize, you can realize it. This book sets out to show you how to bring about the reality by the effective use of the powers of your mind. It takes you on a journey into a new world of infinite positive possibilities where all wishes are granted. Your wish to stop smoking will be granted if you are serious about it.

A PREPARATORY EXERCISE

Now let us begin our quest for success in giving up smoking with a preparatory exercise. The purpose of this is to prepare both the mind and body to the regime of deep relaxation. This will enable you to feel relaxed constantly. It is important to feel relaxed and be relaxed most of the time because with relaxation an individual can do things easily and effectively. With relaxation, your goal of giving up smoking will be accomplished easily and effortlessly. In this way the habit of relaxation will become your everyday reality.

In this exercise we shall go to a world of positive possibilities where all wishes are granted, all goals and desires accomplished and all dreams fulfilled.

Sit down comfortably on a chair or couch and let us start on our journey. Breathe in through your nose. Hold your breath for a mental count from five to zero. 5, 4, 3, 2, 1, z e r o. Now, gently breathe out slowly and go deeper, deeper, deeper and deeper into relaxation. Try to count out the z e r o . . . . as you breathe out and feel the effect. You will feel relaxed immediately but if you do not feel relaxed, continue the breathing exercise until you feel relaxed.

As you are now relaxed, I want you to empty your mind of all doubts, all negative thoughts and mental distortions. Now, I want you to go deeper and deeper into relaxation so that with each breath that you take and at each moment your sense and feeling of relaxation will increase within your mind and body. I want you to learn that from this moment onwards the word **R E L A X** *will bring instant deep relaxation to your mind and body so that whatever situation you are in, wherever you are, you will be absolutely relaxed and in total control, come what may.*

Now, I want you to imagine that you are listening to the sound of my voice or, the sound of your own voice if you have recorded the instructions that I give to you here on your CD or audio tape. Now as I (or you) count the numbers, slowly, down from 10 to zero, you will go ten times more deeply relaxed and you will be relaxed on each and every descending number. Every number down will be a step to peace, tranquillity and total deep relaxation for you. The number now is 10, 9, 8, 7, 6, 5, 4, 3, 2, 1, you are now drifting, shifting, going deeper, deeper, deeper all the way to z e r o.

You are now very, very, very deeply relaxed. I want you to know that some people feel a tingling sensation when they are relaxed by this method, others have a feeling of elation, some others feel very light and weightless, as light as if they can float away. A few other people feel heavy as they are laden with negative thoughts. At this particular moment whatever positive feeling you have is right and proper for you. So stay with your positive feeling as you go deeper, deeper and deeper into relaxation.

Now I want you to come with me for a journey to a new world. This is the world of positive possibilities. It is a world of goodness, a world where you can do good deeds and achieve your goals. You can achieve beneficial results and obtain whatever you want in the world of positive possibilities without harming or undermining anyone.

In this world you can get whatever positive thing you want because whatever positive thing you want is what you get. Every positive wish is granted in this world. Your wish to stop smoking is a positive wish which will be granted in the world of positive possibilities. There is an abundance of good wishes and beneficial things for everyone in this world. In this world all your wishes and desires are fulfilled. You can give up smoking easily, completely, effectively and effortlessly in this world. Now, before we can go to the world of positive possibilities, I want you to become aware of some of the critical health and social reasons for giving up smoking which make this journey to the world of positive possibilities a necessary journey and deliberate on them for a moment before you make the journey.

- *Smoking is poisonous. It poisons and destroys your lungs with tar and nicotine.*
- *Smoking leads to the threat of bronchitis and emphysema.*
- *Smoking causes bad breath, bad cough, irritability, nervousness and tension.*
- *Smoking saps a person's energy, strength and stamina making it difficult for the person to take part in active competitive sports.*
- *Smoking is a very old fashioned, unhealthy and unhygienic habit.*
- *Smoking is now an anti-social habit as it is now forbidden in many public places.*

- *Smoking is a form of self punishment from perverted pleasure in a Sado-Masochistic sort of way since smokers knowingly cause damage to their own bodies in opposition to recognised public health warning.*
- *Smokers are callous. They have no conscience about forcing other people and children around them to become unwilling passive smokers to their own detriment.*
- *The Hollywood image of smokers is very old-hat. The idea which it conjures in the mind of smokers has past its sell by date and use by date. This is a new age, a new millennium of health consciousness.*

As a result of these health and social reasons and many other personal reasons for giving up smoking, you have chosen to go to the world of positive possibilities to give up smoking completely, easily and effectively.

Now, I want you to visualize yourself in the world of positive possibilities. Be there at the count of three to zero. 3,2,1,zero.

You are now in the new world of positive possibilities. You can climb the highest mountain, bungee jump, parachute jump down from the greatest height. You can, accomplish a seemingly impossible feat in the world of positive possibilities. Everything that is positive is possible in this world. Every good wish and positive goal that you want to achieve is easily achievable in this world. Whatever goal you accomplish in the world of positive possibilities will also be accomplished and retained by you in the real world.

Now I want you to visualize yourself as a non-smoker. I want you to stay with the knowledge that in this world, you will accomplish your goal easily and effortlessly. Your positive belief, your optimism and the positive energy which you invest on your positive thoughts of giving up smoking will help you to accomplish your wishes. Now I want you to accomplish your goal of giving up smoking completely in the time that you have in the new world of positive possibilities.

This is your moment, the moment of positive action and positive accomplishment, the moment of healthy living for you. You know what you need to do in order to eliminate smoking from your life completely. Do it now in this opportune moment.

As you are now accomplishing your goal of giving up smoking easily, completely, effectively and effortlessly, I will leave you for a moment for you to complete what you are doing and become a non-smoker easily and effectively. You will be successful in what you are doing and you will accomplish every positive wish or desire that you need to accomplish because every positive wish is granted in the world of positive possibilities and will be retained by you in the real world, they will be actualized by you in the world of actuality.

I will leave you now for you to accomplish your goal, by the time I return you will become a non-smoker, you will be very deeply relaxed and absolutely in control. Go on, do what you have to do in order to accomplish your wish or desire and I will join you in a moment.

(Pause for the reader to perform the exercise)

You are deeply relaxed. You feel peaceful and in control. You have done what you have to do and you have accomplished your goal of giving up smoking and you have done so easily and effortlessly. You are now a non-smoker. Every other positive desire that you have is easily achievable by you from now onwards. Believe it for it is true.

At the count of one to five, you will return to the world of actuality where you will actualize your goal of giving up smoking and every other positive desire that you may have so that they become real and permanent accomplishments for you. You will be very deeply relaxed, confident, positive, very optimistic and in control. These feelings will stay with you and be part of your everyday feelings from this moment onwards. The number now is 1, 2, 3, 4, 5. The number five has been counted. You are welcome to the actual world where you can now actualize your wishes and desires.

Note

You may count the number down to go into relaxation, the higher the number from which you begin your count, the deeper you will relax as follows.

At the count of 10 to zero you will be very deeply relaxed. 10,9,8,7,6,5,4,3,2,1,zero. You are now very deeply relaxed.

Count the numbers upwards to come up, sit up and to open your eyes if they were shut. In general, you may count up or down to perform a specific action in accordance with a specific instruction as follows.

At the count of one to five you will be jumping for joy in the knowledge that you are now a non-smoker. 1,2,3,4,5. You are now a non-smoker.

Where it is necessary to be deeply relaxed and focused to perform a particular action you may count down as follows.

At the count of five to zero you will be deeply relaxed and you will be inside your body to clean out your lungs. Five, four, three, two, one, zero. You are now inside your body. Your job now is to clean out your lungs. (Refer to chapter three for the full details of this powerful exercise).

Now, if you have performed the above preparatory exercise diligently and successfully, the other exercises in this book will become great fun for you because the preparatory exercise sets the pattern of the fun activities in this book. The purpose of the journey to the world of positive possibilities is to underline the role of visualization in mental activities. If you can visualize it, you can realize it, that is, make it real. If you can visualize yourself as a non-smoker in the world of positive possibilities, you will be able to give up smoking easily, completely and effortlessly in the actual world of here and now.

Visualization is a process by which an individual uses positive rational thought to create mental pictures of his or her goals, wishes or desires. The mental pictures help him or her to turn the goals, wishes or desires into reality. In short, visualization is the act of the construction of mind castles.

If you can bring thought and picture together about you giving up smoking and seeing yourself in the picture as a non-smoker, you are conceiving a potent idea, building up something tangible, constructing mind castles. Any wishes, desires, intentions or major goals which you are able to conceive in this way, is easily achievable by you. What you need next is the patience and the right frame of mind to put a rock solid foundation to the castles which you have built in your mind.

However, you can also accomplish your goals, wishes and desire even if you lack the ability to form mental images of what you want. It is sufficient to have an idea of what you want to accomplish and then bring it about through other means which are discussed here. A sound knowledge of the fundamental principles discussed here will help you immensely to accomplish any goal or desire.

THE FUNDAMENTAL PRINCIPLES OF THE MIND TECHNIQUE

Now let us begin our quest for success in giving up smoking right away by examining the fundamental principles of the mind power techniques that are introduced in this book. These principles are the rock solid foundation to your mind castles and a rigid adherence to them will help you to understand what is involved in the use of the power of the mind to make positive changes in your life; a rigid adherence to these principles will enable you to accomplish your goals, wishes and desires. If you understand these principles and act on them rigidly, then you will find that giving up smoking will be fun and easy for you.

In general, you will get what you want for what you want is what you get. The mind techniques which are presented throughout this book are based on the general operation of the human mind in relation to a certain belief of the individual. Thus, in order to understand and master the practical mind techniques for giving up smoking easily and effectively, it is essential that one understands the cardinal principles in our mind technique and apply them generally in one's actions. When this happens constantly the principles will become part of the routine of everyday motor behaviour.

1. The Thought Bricks of the Mind

The thought bricks of the mind can either enhance an individual's power to give up smoking or they can restrict the individual's effort to give up smoking. Thoughts are in the mind and they are the bricks with which we build our impregnable mind castles. In order to build castles in the air or on land, one needs solid and effective thought bricks to lay the foundation of the castle. This principle of mind power stipulates that whatever thoughts you repeat powerfully and often enough will become realities for you. For example, if you are thinking positive thoughts about giving up smoking such as, *I will give up smoking easily and effectively* this will become your reality if the thoughts are powerful and constant in your mind.

The thoughts, whatever they are, which you have in your mind the most often will materialise into reality for you. As in the example above, if you affirm or repeat your thoughts of success in giving up smoking, you will achieve success in giving up smoking steadily, easily and effectively. As mentioned above, if you are thinking positive thoughts about your success in giving up smoking this will become your reality. This applies to any goals, wishes or desires that you may have.

On the other hand, if you are preoccupied with self doubts and negative thoughts about what you want to do, constantly thinking about failures and difficulties, failure and difficulties will become your reality.

The general rule for the application of this principle is to have a positive mental attitude and think positive thoughts so that positive feelings will flow to you, automatically, which will lead you to the achievement of positive results in your life. Thoughts are the bricks of all building structures. Thoughts are in the mind. If your thoughts are all about success you will be successful, if you think mostly about failure, this will become your reality!

If you are always doubting yourself and doubting everything, you must remember that 'doubt' is a thought brick. If 'doubt' is the thought that you have most often in your mind, your 'doubt' will become your reality. Your doubt erases your positive thought and gives you the realisation of failure. If you doubt your ability to give up smoking, if your doubt is the thought that you have most often in your mind, you will prove yourself right by your doubt and fail to give up smoking.

You will get what you think about for what you think about is what you get. You will give up smoking easily and effectively if you think that you will give up smoking, easily and effectively and believe from now onwards that you will give up smoking easily and effectively because this is why you are reading this book. Your belief in the idea of success is a positive thought that stirs your mind to positive efforts and leads you to success. Negative thoughts and self doubts dampen the edge of positive action because they stir your mind away from your chosen objective and thus, lead you to failure and disappointment.

This first fundamental principle of the operation of the mind is vital in everything that we do, the plans and the decisions that we make from day to day. The operation of this first principle is embodied in the functions of the unconscious mind which we will discuss below in this chapter. If what you want to do is not quite clear in your mind, one way to tackle it is to see the problem as a challenge which must be confronted. In this way you will be inspired to investigate the solution and find out more about it.

If your reaction to a problem is negative and you adopt a negative attitude just for the purpose of avoiding the problem or, if you run away completely from the problem, you may find that you will be running away each time you perceive something as a problem; you will not solve any problem by running away from it. Thus, if the supposed problem concerns your goals and aspirations, then it is clear that the goals will not be achieved by running away from them.

2. There is a Limitless Intrinsic Latent Power within Everyone

The power of the human mind is awesome. It can bring great results when it is used in a positive way and it can cause enormous amount of problems, disaster and ruin when used in a negative way. I want you to understand that the power of your mind is potentially unlimited, that is, you have an unlimited potential within you now to accomplish anything you wish and to achieve positive results in your life, including the power to give up smoking even now, easily and effectively.

There is no limit to the power of your mind except those limitations which you wilfully impose on your mind by yourself through negative thoughts. The power of the human mind is ingenious and prodigious. This ingenuity of the human mind enables humans to design sophisticated computers but the power of your mind is much greater than that of the most sophisticated computer because the computer is designed by human mind and it is, by itself, unoriginal.

The power of your mind is there with you throughout your life from the moment of your birth. You can control your entire life with your mind. The magic of success in anything you do is within you. It is within your mind. Your mind is the magic power through which you achieve great success in whatever you do.

The essence of this second principle is that acknowledging the prodigious power of your mind will help you to give up smoking now, easily and effectively, because with increased deep relaxation, the simple mental programmes in this book are easily assimilated in your mind as you read this book.

3. The Principle of Universal Energy

There is a universal energy within everyone. You can channel this energy to your desired goals and aspirations by way of your attitudes. As in the points we made above, positive attitudes toward your goals channel positive energy and negative attitudes and self doubts channel negative energy which leads to lack of fulfilment or disappointment. The energy you put forth and, in the opposite, the energy which you attract to determine how your attitude towards your major goals, your immediate objectives and your life in general relates to what you desire to create for yourself and to the extent, degree or urgency of your desire.

The essential question for you here is to determine what may need to change or evolve within you in order to transform you into a powerfully attractive force of energy so you can bring your goal, objectives or dreams such as give up smoking, now into reality. You can manifest your goals and desires more effectively by channelling positive attitudes towards them with greater expectation of their realization. In other words, the energy of your belief helps to make reality of your goals. Refer also to our first principle above.

In our everyday motor activities, each one of us channels his or her energy as dictated by his or her attitudes, feelings and beliefs in order to obtain the results he or she requires. Although occasionally, unfortunately, it happens that the energy of the individual is channelled negatively and the individual obtains the result that he or she does not require.

The universal energy which is in everyone can also be manifested in a different way in every action of the individual because the individual attracts energy and also radiates energy into the universe by his or her attitudes towards events and situations in his or her life. The energy is manifest in the life of individuals by the state of affairs in their lives such as abundant wealth and prosperity, happiness, success in any venture, destitution, failure in any venture, romantic bliss, confidence, positive feeling, negative feeling and many others.

Also, as in the above examples, other ways in which the energy can be manifested, for example, are in being rich and prosperous, being romantically happy, feeling rejected and alone, feeling inferior, feeling unworthy for success and so forth. All the ways to manifest the energy are within you because the energy is in you. The energy can manifest success, happiness, prosperity and abundance much easier than it can manifest failure and destitution because the natural state of the universe is for happiness, prosperity and abundance.

There is also a central dynamic pure energy force of magnetic power of creativity which is within everyone. The knowledge of this inner magnetic power within you should enable you to change the pattern of your thought and belief system and make them beneficial for you. You can do great things and achieve great goals if you believe that you have a dynamic, pure energy force of magnetic power within you to attract the things you wish in life by your attitudes and your actions.

This is an essential doctrine in depth psychology and it entails the belief that if you think that you can do it, you can. If you believe that you can stop smoking now, then so be it, you can. The force and energy of your belief engenders positive action to realize your wish. This book teaches you to believe that you can, and to always believe that you can, in everything that you do in the general affairs of your life.

You can see quite clearly from what we have been saying here about energy, that success in anything, success in giving up smoking easily and effectively is within you. Success in giving up smoking easily and effectively is a universal energy which is an integral part of your natural limitless, intrinsic latent power within you. Refer to our second principle above. Success and wealth are external expression of abundance but the energy of abundance which causes the success and wealth to manifest in your life is internal. Thus, you can see from this that the magic of success is truly within your actions, your success in giving up smoking now is within you.

4. Every Individual is the Architect of his own Life

Every, adult, individual is responsible for the state of affairs of his or her own life. As a result of an individual's thought patterns in general he or she is responsible for the way and manner he or she makes progress or failure on this planet in respect of the choices and decisions that he or she makes according to how and where his or her thoughts lead to in the execution of a particular action. It is not right for an individual to defend himself or herself for his or her failures and lack of progress at any venture by blaming the state, other people, or by blaming God in appealing to the arguments of determinism, predestination, or fatalism.

You have the freedom to change your life by changing the pattern of your thoughts in making them more positive and beneficial to you. This is an essential principle of mind power. You are the architect of your life and you can change your life by changing the pattern of your thoughts. To profit from this principle, you have to proceed by seeking for ways in which you can take complete control of your life, develop your ideas by making them more beneficial to you, become more and more assertive and self-reliant, and less and less dependent on other people for assistance.

5. Action Is a Positive Expression of Thought

The principle of positive action which we mentioned above is an essential ingredient in a recipe for success in any goal. If it matters to you then the onus is on you to do something about it. If you are truly convinced that you need to give up smoking then you must take action to do so and stop smoking now!

In your actions, you must always act with conviction. If you are giving a positive message to yourself or reading out your own affirmations, you must always act with the conviction that your message is going to be received by your unconscious mind and that your wishes and intentions will be realised, that is, made real.

The essential maxim for action which you must always remember here is that *everything that you believe to be true is true or becomes true for you.* Remember what we said above under the second principle that if you think you can, you can. If you believe that you can do it, you can. No one is ready for success in any venture unless he or she believes that he or she can achieve it.

This is an incontrovertible thesis of mind power. Always endeavour to be enthusiastic in what you do and act with absolute faith in your expectation of success. This part about your expectation is also included in your manifestation of the energy to bring about the desired result.

Remember that we are dealing here with positive action which is provoked by positive thoughts and always avoid the temptation to follow the negative pattern of finger pointing, that is, blaming other people, for example, your partner, the government, tobacco companies, cigarette manufacturers or the supermarkets when things go wrong in your attempt to give up smoking. Take responsibility for your own affairs and do something about it by taking positive action to effect desired changes in your life.

With respect to our first principle which is a cardinal thesis of mind power, it is important to realise that the power of thought is the essence of the mind. The influential French philosopher Rene Descartes (1596–1650) saw this during his great meditations which led him to assert his famous maxim, *Cogito Ergo Sum* (I think, therefore, I am) in his writings, *Discourse on Method* (1637) and *Meditations on First Philosophy* (1641). Descartes saw *thinking* as the indubitable proof of man's existence.

The operation of thinking is a function of the mind. The thinking power of the mind is clearly illustrated in all the deliberations and cogitations which Descartes went through in his meditations and all his other ruminative activities in order to establish the certainty of the *Cogito*. Descartes could have equally said, *Credo Ergo Sum* (I believe, therefore, I am) as your belief is important in arriving at the result you require. Remember that belief is also a thought brick. Refer to the first principle above.

In order to acquire the technique of mind power and be able to build effective mind castles, you must always be able to apply the above fundamental principles of mind power generally in everything you do in your everyday life with respect to your thinking patterns with regard to whatever projects or goals you have. For our own particular purpose in this book, our project or goal is giving up smoking. The fundamental principles mentioned above are applied in the techniques which we discuss in this book together with the secret of how the human mind works.

KEY POINTS TO REMEMBER

- Your thoughts are the bricks for mental constructions. Positive thoughts give solid foundation to your building projects and help you to give up smoking easily and effortlessly. Negative thoughts dampen the edge of positive action, lead to failure, destruction, disappointment and ruin.

- The power of your mind is limitless. Acknowledging this power enables you to know that you can achieve whatever you put your mind to. Thus the magic of success in giving up smoking is truly within you, it is in your positive acknowledgement of the principles we have discussed above in relation to your thoughts about giving up smoking.

- There is a universal energy within you which manifests success or failure according to your thought patterns in relation to your goal of giving up smoking.

- You are the architect of your own life. You have the power to effect changes in your life because it is up to you and not other people.
- Acknowledge that you have the power of a dynamic creative energy force within you which, when recognised, enables you to bring about positive changes in your life.
- The power of your mind is greater than that of the most sophisticated computer because the computer is created by the ingenuity of the human mind.
- Remember that action speaks louder than words and act positively to bring about the changes which you seek.

THE SECRETS OF HOW THE HUMAN MIND WORKS

We can learn a great deal about how the mind works by examining the levels of mental awareness, or the levels of consciousness, if you like. The advantage of this is that by knowing how the mind functions we will be in a better position to direct our thoughts to greater, more beneficial, purposes and achieve the results that we desire. This will help us to programme our mind more effectively with appropriate mental prompts to help us to give up smoking easily, effectively and effortlessly.

An individual's knowledge of how the mind works will enable the individual to appreciate the powers of his or her memory as a facet of the mind and then to achieve the result that he or she desires by using his or her memory to his or her own advantage. We are concerned here with the quality of consciousness in psychical topography.

When you read this book with a serious intention to give up smoking you will find, very quickly, that the deep relaxation exercises and the positive suggestions in the book will become part of your memory which is, in this respect, your unconscious mind. This is where the ideas need to be in order to form part of your motor activity.

The human mind functions at three principal levels. These levels have been clearly recognised within the field of depth psychology, that is, the psychology of the dynamic forces in the interaction between conscious and unconscious mental processes. These levels are more appropriately perceived as levels of mental awareness. They are as follows.

The Conscious Level

This is the level of everyday waking life. You are now reading this book at the conscious level of your mental functioning if you are aware that you are reading this book and know fully well that you are reading it and why you are reading it. The conscious level of mental function is the level of operation when one is awake and so at this level one is able to reason, criticise and control voluntary action. Your decision to give up smoking is made at this level.

The Preconscious Level

This is the level of latent ideas which are capable of becoming conscious at anytime. For instance, there were some things which happened to you last year, last month, yesterday or last week and some other things which you caused to happen last week, yesterday, last month or last year in so far as their occurrence was the direct result of your own action.

As I have now got your undivided attention because you are listening to me, attentively, at this moment in reading this book, your mind is not concentrating on the events of yesterday, last week, last month or last year because it is occupied with the events of the moment in listening to what I am saying to you.

However since I have now provoked you or stirred up your mind by mentioning the events of yesterday, last week, last month or last year, the flow of thoughts of those events may now come to your mind without difficulty because they have been triggered by my reference to them.

The memories that have now been triggered by my reference to them are said to be at the preconscious level of mental functioning because they are latent memories which are at the threshold of consciousness. They are not being used at any particular moment, though they are not forgotten.

The Unconscious Level

This level was first investigated as a way to understand the power of the mind and the basis for the treatment of mental disorders by the Viennese neurologist and physiologist, Sigmund Freud (1856–1939), founder of psychoanalysis. It is the most confused and confusing level of mental functioning. For our purpose here the theory of the unconscious consists of the following.

- The idea of the inaccessibility of mental items to consciousness due to their repression.
- The belief that such mental items which are inaccessible are, at the same time, causally active. Unconscious items have the power to affect the individual by giving rise to psychoneurotic symptoms and other puzzling or embarrassing behaviours whose origins have escaped the individual's consciousness because of their repression which makes them inaccessible.
- The belief that unconscious materials belong to a general psychical system of unconsciousness to which all unconscious materials inhere. This general psychical system is described by Freud as the *system unconscious*.
- Memories which are stored in the unconscious remain there permanently until released by the individual.

However, for the purpose of our understanding of mind power, your own unconscious mind is the simple and uncomplicated part of your mental awareness at which your mind is deeply relaxed and is totally uncluttered by bias, criticism, self doubt, tension, general disbelief, etc. At this level the mind faithfully records, reproduces and controls the entire programme of an individual's life.

In this respect, every experience of an individual's life, every feeling, reaction, emotion, etc. is recorded in the unconscious level of his mind and can be reproduced during moments of deep relaxation. The unconscious is seen, in this sense, as the reservoir of everything that happens in an individual's life and everything that constitutes the individual's personality. It is the totality of an individual's character and attitudes, the storehouse of all memory, and the centre of the individual's habits. I have described this view of the unconscious elsewhere as the *container theory of the mind* (Antony Maurice-Nneke 2003).

In his *Collected Works, Volume 8,* the Swiss psychiatrist, Carl Gustav Jung (1875–1961), founder of the Society of Analytical Psychology and former sidekick of Sigmund Freud, describes the unconscious as a "receptacle of all memories."

With respect to giving up smoking the unconscious level of the mind functions in an automatic way, recording and reproducing the events of an individual's life. All beliefs, thoughts, feelings, etc, are stored or recorded in the unconscious, the everlasting receptacle and these are reproduced automatically in the individual's thoughts and motor actions.

For example, if a person has negative thoughts and believes that he or she might fail with his or her goal of giving up smoking such belief is stored or recorded in the person's unconscious and reproduced in his or her motor actions. Such a person will not take a positive action to give up smoking because he or she believes that such action will be a failure. Thus, failure will become his or her reality because he or she thinks about failure. In other words, a person who has a negative attitude towards his or her goal will find that the negative attitude will be recorded in his or her unconscious mind and failure will become his or her reality. Refer to our first fundamental principle discussed above.

On the other hand, if the individual has positive beliefs about himself or herself, his or her goals and aspirations about giving up smoking and feeling fit, healthy and energetic, these are what will be recorded in the unconscious and they will come true for him or her in his or achievement of positive results in his or her intentions. The unconscious level controls involuntary action and it is very receptive and active during sleep and in waking state. Remember the first principle of mind power, what you think of most often becomes your reality. This is because what you think of most often is what is recorded in the unconscious mind.

At the unconscious level all rational thought are suspended. Thus at this level, the mind does not reason, analyse, or criticize. Instead, all thinking processes which are carried out at the conscious level are stored up and played back in the unconscious. Thus, when ideas and beliefs are recorded in the unconscious, whether false or true beliefs, the mind retains them automatically and the ideas, beliefs, thoughts, or feelings are acted out by the individual in motor activity.

This is how your thoughts become your reality. This is how it is possible for you to give up smoking easily and effectively. The positive ideas contained in this book, which we programme into your unconscious mind are the ones which would be retained by your unconscious mind to be acted out in your motor activity!

With respect to this power of the unconscious, you can see clearly from what we have said here that when positive ideas about success in giving up smoking are recorded in the unconscious, the individual automatically thinks positively about achieving success in giving up smoking and in whatever venture he or she engages in.

However, when negative ideas are recorded in the unconscious in relation to the ideas of the subject or venture, the individual shies away from the subject or venture and procrastinates and vacillates about the right things to do or the most appropriate goals to have and ends up with nothing because he or she is unable to decide.

As a matter of information, the term *unconscious,* as described above and used throughout this book, is the correct name for what you, probably, know as the 'subconscious'. The term 'subconscious' implies an inferior state and does not give an adequate description of the dynamics of mental processes. On the contrary, the unconscious is the most powerful force in the dynamics of mental functions. If you wish to know more about the unconscious, refer to my more elaborate book on the subject, *The Psychodynamics of the Unconscious* (2003).

The Supraconscious Level

There is a fourth level of mental awareness known as the *supraconscious* level. This is responsible for direct knowing and it functions independent of ordinary thought processes. It is utilised for extrasensory perception (ESP). ESP is a term which is used to describe four areas of mind power. These are the powers of clairvoyance, precognition, psychokinesis (also known as telekinesis), and telepathy.

Clairvoyance is the power to specifically perceive or know an event or object that is out of the natural range of human knowledge or perception, without the use of ordinarily recognised means of human knowledge or perception. *Precognition* is the power of knowledge of future events in advance of their occurrence without deducing their occurrence from available data. *Psychokinesis* (PK) or *Telekinesis* (TK) is the power to use the mind to cause motion and changes in external objects. *Telepathy,* also known as thought transference, is the power of direct mental communication between two persons who may not necessarily be at close quarters.

A person who is adept in the use of any of these powers of the mind is usually described, as *psychic* and the four areas of mind power constitute what is called *psi* (referring to psychic power). However, the term *psi* is also the name of the 23rd letter in the Greek alphabet. This term is usually employed in theories, equations, and experiments to denote an unknown quantity as opposed to what is given or postulated.

Thus, to the world of natural science psi, as denoted by the four areas of mind power given above, is still an unknown quantity despite decades of psychical research by eminent parapsychologists in Britain and the USA. But this is not totally surprising because natural science is slow to open up to ideas outside its limited boundary and it is opposed to the existence of the mind. Many scientists, as scientists, disdain the idea of the psychical or the mental. They believe that everything is physical. As individuals, however, they may admit to themselves that mind exists otherwise they make no sense when they use the expression 'I have a mind of my own'.

Many people today still scoff at an individual's manifestation of any psi power. For example, before his resignation from the International Psychoanalytic Association, Carl Gustav Jung showed his psychokinetic powers to Sigmund Freud but, as a man who believed solidly in science, Freud scoffed at it, described Jung as a mystic and questioned the scientific validity of ESP and mysticism. Even today in the new millennium ESP power is still looked at with disapproval in some quarters. Thus those who possess some of the ESP powers described above only advertise their craft in the back pages of astrological publications and esoteric magazines.

Some people are very sceptical and cynical. They doubt that the clairvoyants possess any powers of vision and still regard them as charlatans. Some other people wear the 'It's not scientific' (INS) cloak. This is an imaginary cloak of intellectual smugness which confers an illusory sense of superiority to those who wear it while, at the same time, it betrays their lack of understanding. Such people find it difficult to give credit to what they are unable to understand or explain scientifically.

Thus, they embarrass themselves by seeking refuge in their own limitations of knowledge.

I am not saying that you should endorse the psychics if you have doubts about their claims. Far from it, I believe that if you have genuine doubt, as an educated person, your doubt should provoke you to investigate the topic of doubt further, if only for the purpose of proving that you are right in your suspicions. I am saying, very strongly, that you should only doubt any claim if you have constructive arguments to refute the claim.

I firmly believe that a truly educated person is one who has an open mind to the things he or she does not understand and cannot explain. As part of our on-going epistemological enquiry, any speckle or atom of suspicion, doubt or scepticism on a particular subject of enquiry should give us the green light or the impetus for further investigation in our search for knowledge and certainty in the particular subject of enquiry. This is positive scepticism which leads to further investigation, knowledge and certainty as opposed to plain, naive, doubt which perpetuates ignorance.

You must always remember that until one's investigations, things do not become rubbish, silly or stupid just because one lacks the experience or the intellectual ability to understand them! Always remember that what you know is not all there is to know in heaven and earth as William Shakespeare cautions here.

> "There are more things in heaven and earth, Horatio,
> Than are dreamt in your philosophy."
>
> (William Shakespeare, *Hamlet* Act 1, Scene 5)

KEY POINTS TO REMEMBER

There are four levels of mental action

- The Conscious level is the level of everyday waking life, the level at which you are reading this book now.

- The Preconscious level is the level of latent memories which can be recalled at any moment without difficulty.
- The Unconscious level is the level of memories which have been repressed and have become inaccessible to the individual.
- The Supraconscious level is the level of great natural creativity, inspirational work and the power of the mind for extrasensory perception.

BELIEF AS AN ESSENTIAL INGREDIENT FOR GIVING UP SMOKING

Belief, like action, is an essential ingredient in a recipe for success in anything you do. It is an attitude of mind which encompasses everything you do in relation to the objectives you which to accomplish.

There is an enormous power in believing. A man or woman can achieve a seemingly impossible goal, perform the greatest feat and achieve a personal best (PB) performance in competitive sports when he or she believes in the possibility of accomplishing the goal. A person's belief or conviction has an effect on the way he lives his life because it can make the difference between success and failure. You can give up smoking now, easily and effortlessly if you strongly believe that you can. Remember the positive possibilities in your journey to the new world in our preparatory exercise at the beginning of this chapter and have the idea of the possibility of success in your mind always.

Belief can be positive or negative. Each form of belief affects the individual differently. A positive belief is a detergent to doubt. A positive belief that you will give up smoking now stirs your mind to positive action and enables you to give up smoking easily, effectively and effortlessly. A belief that you would not be able to give up smoking, that it is all a waste of time, is a negative belief. This form of belief blunts the edge of positive action and leaves you incapable of accomplishing your objectives. A negative belief in relation to your goal leads disastrously to failure.

A negative belief fans the flames of doubts and panders to idleness. Both positive and negative beliefs are ways of channelling your energy to your objectives or goals. The positive energies bring success to you while the negative energies bring failure and disappointment to you. In order to understand this properly, you must refer to the principles of mind power which we discussed above at the beginning of this chapter.

YOU MUST HAVE TOTAL BELIEF AND FAITH IN YOURSELF

In another sense belief is an attitude of mind which encompasses everything you do in relation to what you wish to achieve. The power of belief is in its usage; it is not something which you possess and leave at home in your briefcase or something which you leave in a box, cupboard, or in your pocket. Belief is something about you which lies in the power within you in expressing your attitudes in everything you do to achieve your objectives. Belief, like confidence, is the way you carry yourself strongly, forcefully, in your actions, attitudes and behaviours from day to day.

There is a strong sense in what I have said above, in which belief refers to absolute trust or confidence. This is the sense in which we use the word **belief** in this book. It is the sense in which we say 'I believe in God' or the sense in which we may say to someone that, 'You must have total belief in yourself'.

This sense of belief is like **faith,** an absolute, confident trust in the truth, value, efficacy, or worthiness of the ideas or plans which you hold on a given project. Belief is, in this sense, very essential for success because it enhances your powers of persistence. You must understand in this sense that no one is ready for success in anything until he or she believes that he or she can acquire it.

You must have absolute faith and trust in yourself and in what you are doing in order to succeed in your venture. Belief is the opposite of doubt. When you have belief you are able to pursue your goals without doubting your ability to succeed in them In order to understand this much better you must refer to our discussions above on the principles of mind power.

What is pertinent for our present purpose of giving up smoking is that those beliefs which a person, mistakenly, takes as knowledge are recorded permanently in the unconscious mind. These affect the person's attitude in relation to the things that matter in his or her life. A false and negative belief in relation to giving up smoking and the achievement of success will cause a person to have twisted ideas about giving up smoking. These twisted ideas must be eradicated and replaced with positive ideas backed up with belief for the individual to achieve success with the goal of giving up smoking or with any other goal in a chosen field of endeavour.

Belief is the essential ingredient in a recipe for success in whatever you do, you must have total belief in yourself and in whatever venture you wish to embark on in order to succeed in it. You must have an unwavering, rock solid, absolute belief in yourself and in your ability to give up smoking easily and effortlessly. Some people start by doubting themselves. They ask, "What if it fails?" They convince themselves that this is an appropriate question. Remember, if you have failure in your mind, that is what you will get. If you are thinking of failure, that will be your reality. Endeavour to think about success in whatever you do, in your goals and aspirations, so that success will be your reality. Refer to the fundamental principles which we discussed above.

KEY POINTS TO REMEMBER

- Belief is the essential ingredient in a recipe for success in any venture.

- You must have total belief, a rock solid, absolute faith in yourself in order to be successful in whatever you do.
- Belief is the opposite of doubt. When you have belief you pursue your goals without doubts about your chances of success.
- Remember that no one is ready for success in anything until he or she believes that he or she is capable of achieving success.

HOW TO ELIMINATE THE NEGATIVE POWER OF SELF DEFEAT

Remember that belief is the opposite of doubt. Do not defeat yourself by doubting yourself before you start. Do not place unwanted barriers on your path to success through relentless but unnecessary doubts. Self doubt shows insecurity, lack of self esteem and lack of faith in your ability to achieve success with your goal. If you lack faith in yourself how would you expect others to have faith in your?

The way to get out of the negative, defeatist, thinking trap is to break down the negative thought patterns that restrict you from making essential progress in your chosen field. Whenever negative thoughts flow to your mind in relation to your ability to give up smoking, you must start to cancel them out by thinking positive thoughts about the possibility of attaining your desire of being a non-smoker easily and effectively. Remember your journey to the world of positive possibilities. When you visualize your success you will be able to realize it, that is, make it real.

You will find that each time you introspect about the good things that have happened to you in your life, all the goals you have achieved in the past till now, or think positive thoughts about your life in general, think about the positive effects of giving up smoking easily, effectively and being a non-smoker right now! If you are unable to visualize, then endeavour to think strong, powerful thoughts about your success in anything you do so that success will be your reality.

You will find that as you concentrate your thoughts in this way, positive feelings will flow, automatically, to you. *Think positive thoughts and positive feelings will flow to you, automatically.* It works every time. Try it **NOW** and see what happens. Go on try it now even as you read this book. You will feel positive instantly. Remember, if you think you can, you will succeed. Think about the positive possibilities of giving up smoking easily, effectively and effortlessly and you will give up smoking.

If you are disagreeing with me at this moment and saying to yourself that you have not achieved anything in your life, you would be very wrong! Do not be too quick to condemn yourself or to argue and disagree with me because this is the basis of insecurity. Think about it seriously. You may have been quick to disagree with what I have said here because there is anxiety in your life at the moment or because you have been using the word 'achieve' in a negative sense.

You have definitely achieved successes in your life. Take a deep breath, relax and look back with confidence and you will find plenty of successes in your life. Most important of all, remember that you have conquered some obstacles in life and got over certain difficulties in life to be where you are now.

In addition, you are now making plans for your success with the goal of giving up smoking easily and effectively. You have started on this plan by reading this book and you will finish what you start; remember the five principles above. When you believe in yourself and think positive thoughts in the way that I am teaching you here, things will happen for you as you wish them to happen. They happen because you are making them happen by the effective use of the power within you.

Begin **today** to develop a different sense of value about yourself, self-worth, time, energy, work and your desire to give up smoking. Begin from now onwards to evaluate yourself positively, to project a positive self image. Begin now to believe in yourself for this will help you to give up smoking easily and effectively.

If you hold negative beliefs about yourself, about the idea of success in giving up smoking, then the thing to do now is to change your pattern of beliefs and begin today to see that success is within your grasp because the magic power of success is within you. Start from now to believe in yourself and you will easily see a way out of any difficult situation.

Start from now to believe that there is **always** a way out of any problem. Begin now to do things differently from the way you have done in the past. This is what making a change is about, doing something new or at least different from before. Start from today to believe that life is full of doors of opportunities opening up for you. Believe it for it is true.

Use your mind positively to find a way out of any current problem which you may have. If you want to make progress in the face of mounting problems, remember to *always look on the bright side of life* and then do something new or, at least, different from what you have done in the past. This book offers you something different, new methods of dealing with problems through mental action. Your mind is the very fertile womb through which all the thoughts for positive mental constructions are incubated and hatched.

KEY POINTS TO REMEMBER

- Remember that whenever you think positive thoughts about yourself, your goals and aspirations, you will find that positive feelings flow to you automatically.

- Always look on the bright side of life because irrational negativism dampens the spirits of positive action.
- Remember that belief is a detergent to doubt.

POSITIVE STRATEGIES TO ENHANCE YOUR SUCCESS IN GIVING UP SMOKING

How to Guard Against Negatives in General

In order for an individual to achieve success in whatever venture he or she embarks on, he or she must endeavour to guard himself or herself against negative influences. Some negative influences may be of the individual's own making. Where this is the case, it is often difficult for the individual to recognise the negative influences upon him or her because people, in general, do not perceive themselves as impediments to their own progress.

Other negative influences may be the result of the activities of the negative people with whom an individual associates, that is, the company he or she keeps or the negative environment in which he or she works in or lives in. If you live or work with people who influence you to smoke against your wishes you must begin from now to tell them that you are now a non-smoker. To gather the confidence to take control and dispel the negative influence of other people, make the journey to the world of positive possibilities now. Refer to the beginning of this chapter.

Whatever the negative influences in an individual's life are, and whatever form they have been derived, the individual must be able to recognise these negative influences and eliminate them in order to feel mentally free to entertain positive thoughts about success. This is particularly relevant in giving up smoking because friends and associates may attempt to deter one from a chosen purpose by their negative vibrations. Stick to your plans and you will be successful in giving up smoking easily and effectively.

An individual must become aware of his or her own will power and remember, always, that the magic of success is truly within him or her. The recognition of this will alert the person to the power of the unconscious mind and thus help him or her to eliminate negatives from his or her thoughts in relation to the goal of giving up smoking. An individual must become aware that negative thoughts will affect him or her if such thoughts are allowed to take hold in his or her unconscious mind.

In this respect it is most appropriate for an individual to avoid the association of people whose company drain the individual's energy psychically and makes the individual feel low, depressed or unhappy in some ways. If you wish to give up smoking now, easily and effortlessly you must avoid the association of negative people who constantly make you feel bad by forcing you to smoke against your will.

To eliminate such negatives influences a person must master the five principles we have discussed above because a sound knowledge of the five principles is a detergent to negative influences. An individual must also seek the company of people in whose association he or she gets an uplift, people who inspire him or her with confidence and make him or her feel good about himself or herself, or people whose achievements he or she admires and seeks to emulate.

Confront Your Fear to Conquer It

Do not be afraid of success. Some individuals are afraid of success but they convince themselves that they are afraid of failure so they fail to act on opportunities that come their way and, thus, fail to accomplish their objective just as they fail to recognize their own negative thinking. Do not be afraid of success. Do not think that you will fail because if you think of failure, failure will become your reality. Remember the fundamental principles discussed in this chapter. If you are thinking of failure, this will become your reality. You must confront your fear and conquer it.

Fear is an impediment to your goal of giving up smoking and it can be manifested by your vacillation, procrastination and doubting your own ability to succeed in giving up smoking. Sometimes people vacillate and procrastinate because they are uncertain of what to do and this uncertainty may be the result of insecurity which, also, leads to fear. Thus, here, there is a circle which can be a vicious circle in certain individual circumstances.

Fear is a hindrance to success in general and must be confronted for the individual to succeed in a chosen goal. Many sporting personalities and teams have lost competitions because they were afraid of the opponents. Think about success in giving up smoking so that success will become your reality.

Fear is ordinarily an emotional or physiological response to a consciously recognized source of danger. The normal response takes the form of voluntary avoidance of the feared object. However, fear can occur unconsciously and may be employed by a person in a defence mechanism as a pretext to exculpate the failure to act in a certain way. Instances of such defences may occur if the person concerned has convinced himself or herself that he or she is afraid of attempting to give up smoking.

In such circumstances, such a person, then, automatically avoids anything that will lead him or her to attempt to give up smoking. Thus, he or she never takes part in any ventures to do with giving up smoking because of his or her fear of failure. The effect of such fear is that it destroys positive thoughts about giving up smoking, weakens the power of reflection on the advantages of giving up smoking and discourages positive effort in relation to giving up smoking in general.

Remember our discussions above about the powers of the unconscious mind. You will understand from this that fear will have a very dangerous effect on a person's attempt to give up smoking. As we have described above, if a person is afraid of doing something, the natural response is to avoid the object or topic of fear. In doing so, the fear and its avoidance are retained in the unconscious and, as a result of this, the fear is perpetuated by the person in an automatic way.

Thus when a person gives expression to fear in the form of negative and destructive thoughts about giving up smoking, he or she is very likely to experience the result of the fear in the form of destructive repercussions. The negative thoughts are retained in the unconscious and this becomes part of his or her general attitude, response, reaction and behavioural traits in relation to giving up smoking. Such a person becomes a very negative, fearful, cowardly person lacking courage and moral fibre to make a definite decision to give up smoking and stick with the decision or to embark on anything worthwhile because of fear.

If a person wishes to give up smoking and, at the same time, has fear of giving up smoking, fear that he or she might fail to give up smoking, then it is clear from our discussion of fear that such a person has a psychological conflict. Such conflict is necessary in the development of neurotic anxiety and all those seemingly simple problems that blight an individual's enjoyment of everyday life. For a fuller discussion of **conflicts** in the development of psychoneurotic problems, refer to my book, *The Psychodynamics of the Unconscious* (2003).

How to Deal With the Effects of Stress, Anxiety and Depression (SAD)

The effects of stress, anxiety, and psychological depression can be very damaging to a person's personality. They can lead to apathy, lack of confidence and very low self-esteem. Thus stress, anxiety and psychological depression bring about destructive negative attitudes which are barriers to progress in a chosen goal such as giving up smoking. Indeed, with some individuals stress, anxiety and psychological depression may be the cause of their smoking problem.

The people who suffer from anxiety problems, those who live or work in stressful environment or those who suffer from psychological depression, find it difficult to live in a healthy way. They may smoke constantly for comfort and thus may convince themselves that smoking helps them to feel relaxed. The reality is that excessive smoking for comfort makes the individual tense, nervous and irritable. This is the effect of the mass of tar and nicotine in the individual's metabolic system. I use the term, *psychological depression*, to refer to an emotional problem of interpersonal relations which leads to a deep feeling of unhappiness and total inadequacy. This is distinguished from *organic depression* which is the result of some injury to the brain.

The unhappiness involved in psychological depression is often manifested in the individual's need to resort to food, alcohol or cigarette as a means of comfort, but it is in reality a means of escape for the individual, that is, the individual is running away from the need to confront the problem. For some other people suffering from stress, anxiety and psychological depression, food, alcohol and cigarettes offer a means of denial of the their problem by acting as a defence mechanism since for such people, the enjoyment of food, alcohol and cigarettes give the illusory feeling that everything is fine with them, that they are relaxed as I have mentioned above.

A person who suffers from psychological depression has certain underlying psychological problems which make him or her feel very low and unhappy. As I have mentioned above, where certain underlying feeling of unhappiness exists in an individual's life, it is often difficult for the individual to attend positively to a goal such as giving up smoking. Such a person, usually, resorts to negative attitudes such as self-pity, excuses, etc. Stress, anxiety and psychological depression are barriers to giving of smoking because they prevent an individual from concentrating fully on the tasks and exercises that are conducive to the goal of giving up smoking easily, effectively and effortlessly.

To find out whether you are properly attuned in your mind to the goal of giving up smoking easily and effectively, you must examine your private life thoroughly and answer the following questions truthfully and honestly to yourself.

- Do you have stress and anxiety in your life?
- Do you suffer from episodes of depression in your life?
- Are you depressed now?
- Are you prone to destructive negative thoughts most of the time?
- Do you live with people or a person who abuse you, bully or beat you?

Do not be troubled because it is not an intelligent test or an aptitude test. However, if you are frank and sincere in your answers you will find out more about your own personal issues and then be able to make improvements as necessary. If you admit to anxiety and depression, it is best that you deal with these problems first by consulting your own physician who may be able to recommend a psychotherapist. You will find that the solution of the problems will enable you to concentrate more on your chosen venture of giving up smoking, easily and effectively. Here are the rest of the exercises which you must now administer to yourself before we proceed to our exercises for giving up smoking.

EXAMINING YOUR LEVEL OF STRESS, ANXIETY, AND DEPRESSION

Recognising the SAD Effect

A person who is afflicted with stress, anxiety, and depression is very usually a sad person. The sadness is often noticed in his or her behaviour and attitudes by other people with whom he or she comes into contact such as family, friends or working colleagues. By coincidence, the first letters of the words *stress, anxiety, depression,* spell out **SAD** just as in the case of the condition known as *seasonal affective disorder.* Find out whether this **SAD** effect is part of your personal issue or whether it is implicated in your behaviour or in your everyday attitudes towards people or things and events around you.

Answer the following questions in your own way but truthfully to yourself. If you choose to answer just 'YES' or 'NO' to any of the questions, let your 'YES' or 'NO' be represented by what happens to you most of the time with the situation described in the particular question. Do not say 'It depends on . . . ' as an answer to any of the question because we are dealing with general situations, not contextual or particular circumstances or situations in your life.

However, if you choose to answer 'YES' or 'NO' to any questions, be particularly careful that you do not answer 'YES' and 'NO' to the same question. For example, in the third question below, if your general attitude is to interrupt when people talk with you, then your answer to the question would be 'YES'. If you are unable to decide what your answer to a particular question should be and if you think that the questions are designed to annoy you or make you reveal your deep secrets, this is indicative that there are, indeed, certain underlying problems in your life.

If any of the questions make you say to yourself, "Everyone does that," you will be wrong because you do not **know** *everyone* however much you may wish to think that you do! At the best, all the people you know may be doing that, but all the people you know are not, strictly speaking, *everyone,* they are just *some* people that do whatever is implied in the question. In matters such as those in our questions, it is best to speak for yourself always but not for everyone.

By saying to yourself or to others that "Everyone does that" you are, unconsciously, employing the psychological defence mechanism of *rationalisation*. You are trying to make your unwanted behaviour or habit 'fit' with what you think everyone does, that you are the same as everyone. This is to show that all is well with you since your habit, action or behaviour is in accord with public habit, action or behaviour. By doing this, you are defending yourself already before anyone has accused you of anything!

Just relax and remember that your name does not appear anywhere on the questions. They are general, questions and you are reading them alone in your own privacy and giving the answers to yourself. There is, therefore, nothing to be alarmed about. Now, read carefully and answer all the questions sincerely and honestly to yourself in your own way.

EXAMINING THE LEVEL OF ANXIETY IN YOUR LIFE

1. *In general, are you a negative or a positive person?*
2. *Would you describe yourself as an optimist or a pessimist?*
3. *Do you often interrupt when someone is talking to you?*
4. *Are you always in a rush but really not accomplishing anything?*
5. *Can you wait your turn patiently?*
6. *Do you usually hide your feelings?*
7. *Do you do lots of things at once?*
8. *Would you describe yourself as a difficult person?*
9. *Do you often feel you want to burst into tears?*
10. *Do you bite your nails?*
11. *Do you have any nervous twitches?*
12. *Do you find it hard to concentrate or make decisions?*
13. *Do you often feel irritable, snappy, or unfriendly?*
14. *Do you often find yourself eating when you are not hungry?*
15. *Do you regularly drink or smoke to calm your nerves?*

16. *Do you sleep badly?*
17. *Have you lost interest in sex?*
18. *Do you feel increasingly gloomy and suspicious of other people?*
19. *Do you blush when people look straight at you?*
20. *Are you a calm person who is not easily upset?*
21. *Can you sit still without fidgeting?*
22. *Can you keep your cool when your plans fail to work?*
23. *Are you afraid of the dark?*
24. *Are you afraid of death? Cancer? Blood? Heights?*
25. *Have you ever used tranquillisers to calm your nerves?*
26. *Are you on tranquillisers now?*
27. *Do you care about making an impression by what you do?*
28. *Do you often stop to examine your motives?*
29. *Do you care much about what other people think of you?*
30. *Do you seem to have more than your share of bad luck?*
31. *Do you feel usually depressed when you wake up in the morning?*
32. *In general are you satisfied with your life so far?*
33. *Do you often suffer from loneliness?*
34. *Do you consider your future as quite bright?*

EXAMINING WHETHER YOU ARE IN CONTROL

1. *Are there some habits of yours that you would like to break but cannot?*
2. *Do you make your decisions in spite of what other people concerned have to say?*
3. *If something you have planned goes wrong, do you usually admit it is your own fault rather than blame it on bad luck?*
4. *Do you often feel that you are the victim of other peoples plots or outside forces which you cannot control?*
5. *Are you always persuaded into action by what other people say?*
6. *Do you believe that it is possible for a person to change his/her personality?*

7. *Do you reckon that you can do things as well as other people?*

8. *Do you spend more of your time thinking about success or failure?*

9. *Do you sometimes think about yourself as a failure?*

10. *Are there many things about yourself that you would like to change if you could?*

11. *Are you bothered by other people's criticisms of your personality or your actions?*

12. *Do you often think that other people are better liked than yourself?*

13. *Can you honestly say that you rarely feel ashamed of anything you have done?*

14. *Do you often set your aspirations low in order to avoid disappointments?*

15. *Do you try to do things immediately rather than put them off until later?*

16. *Do you always try to finish the things you start?*

17. *Do you always tend to be jealous or envious of the success of other people?*

18. *Have you ever felt that you would really like to kill someone?*

19. *If someone does you a bad turn do you usually ignore it?*

20. *Do you sometimes get so annoyed that you break crockery or throw things around the house?*

21. *Do you usually resort to tantrums as your only way of attracting attention to ourselves?*

EXAMINING YOUR POWER TO PROJECT YOURSELF POSITIVELY

1. *Do you usually seek revenge when someone hurts you in any way?*

2. *Would you rather agree with what someone had said so as to avoid an argument?*

3. *Do you feel that if someone is rude to you it is best to ignore them and let the occasion pass?*

4. *Do you often make sarcastic remarks about other people in their presence or behind their back?*

5. *Do you tolerate negative or discouraging influences which you can easily avoid?*

6. *If you have been waiting on a queue for a long time and someone came in and went straight to the front of the queue would you do something about it?*

7. *Do you usually put yourself second in matters relating to your family?*

8. *Do you believe that it is necessary to fight for your rights or else you lose them?*

9. *Do you complain if something you purchased in good faith turns out to be a fake?*

10. *You were ignored in a store. Do you act to attract attention or just leave quietly?*

KEY POINTS TO REMEMBER

- Always guard against negative thoughts and endeavour to be positive at all times.
- Endeavour to eliminate the SAD effect, if any, from your life.
- Take control of your life and project yourself positively.

CHAPTER TWO

The Goal and a Plan of Action for Giving Up Smoking

You will get what you want for what you want is what you get

A prime requisite for success is to determine accurate goals or objectives. This is accomplished by establishing what you regard as your major and minor goals. A major goal may be something which would bring a major change in an individual's life or it may be those long range objectives which an individual hopes to achieve within a long period of time, for example, say within three years, five years, ten years, etc. as in the expressed desire, *By this time in five years I will be a billionaire!*

A minor goal should be the short term range of objectives which a person seeks to achieve this month, within the next three months or six months as the case may be. In certain cases there may be a series of minor goals leading to the fulfilment of a major goal.

In our case, the goal to stop smoking now is a shot term goal because it needs to be fulfilled now. However, it can be a major goal for an individual if attaining the desired smoke free life style involves a long term plan or if the attainment of the desired non-smoker status would bring a major change in the individual's life as a whole. Nevertheless, the time element

'*Now*' is indicative of the urgency of the wish and the necessity to accomplish it immediately or within a short time.

HOW TO FORMULATE THE GOAL TO GIVE UP SMOKING

For our own specific purpose here to stop smoking now, a well formulated goal must have the following characteristics.

1. The Goal must be specific and Clearly Defined

Every individual has a series of ambitions, desires, hopes, needs, wants, wishes. These, initially, are not goals but each one of your ambitions, desires, hopes, needs, wants, or wishes can become your major goal or minor goal as the case may be from the moment the particular ambition, desire, hope, need, want, or wish is isolated from the rest and made the central focus of your mental and physical energy, that is the energy required for your mental and physical efforts to achieve the objective. Refer to our third principle discussed above in the first part of this book.

To isolate any objective and make it into a goal you must put your series of ambitions, desires, hopes, needs, wants, and wishes into a scale of relative preference and deal with the one that is most pressing, most urgent, or most easily attainable. You must deal with the economic consideration involved. For example, the most pressing and most urgent objective may not be the most easily achievable.

Something becomes a goal for an individual when, after all the work of consideration and deliberations in evaluating its merits and disadvantages, the individual isolates it from the series of other ambitions, desires, needs, wants, or wishes, etc, which are open to him or her, and then focus all mental and physical energies towards achieving that particular objective.

For example in order to achieve the goal of giving up smoking easily and effortlessly, the individual has to focus his or her attention on the health and integrity of his or her body, the need to get back the strength and stamina which was lost through smoking, the need for positive thoughts about himself or herself and his or her ability to succeed in the goal. He or she must have self belief. Remember that no one is ready for success in any goal unless he or she believes that he or she is capable of achieving success in the goal.

Defining your goal clearly means that it should be properly distinguished from your range of other interests, ambitions, desires, need, wants, and wishes. It also means that the road to the fulfilment of your goal must be clearly mapped out showing what you ought to do, the length of time you have set aside to do it, and how you are to do what you ought to do in order to achieve the goal. In other words, defining the goal entails part of the action plan to accomplish the goal

2. The Goal must involve new Behaviour or new Activity and a Plan of Action

When a goal is clearly formulated the formulation will include the definition of what the goal entails, and the plan of action that would bring the goal about. The execution of this plan must involve the individual in new behaviours, doing things which he or she has not done before or things which he or she is not doing at the moment.

Thus in order to achieve the goal the individual must be actively involved in a new form of activity or behaviour. In order to give up smoking easily and effortlessly the individual must start with a new course of action such as the regime of mental action which this book brings to you.

3. The Goal must be Positive and Realistic

If your goals are positive they become easy for you to fulfil and you will fulfil them much quicker if they are realistic. The goal to give up smoking is a positive goal for an individual in respect of the improvement to the person's health. The person gains also in strength, energy, stamina and vitality which an individual derives from the cessation of the debilitation effect of smoking.

4. The Goal must be Available

If you have taken great care and thought to formulate and define your goal you will see, easily, that if the goal is within your reaches, it will be attainable effortlessly. At one of my *Self Help Workshops* a gentleman participant stated that his goal was to own a Rolls Royce car. As he had no savings and investments and was earning only £100 per week from his employment at the time you can see, quite clearly, that the stated goal was not available to him at the time.

There is every reason to say that, although the goal was a positive one in so far as it was forward looking, it was indeed an unrealistic goal in respect of his financial position at the time. It is obvious that in view of his financial position the desire (for it was only a desire for him at the time not a goal yet!) for a Rolls Royce car will take an awfully long time to be accomplished. Thus, his immediate goal would, more appropriately, be a change of employment to a higher wage structure.

The goal to give up smoking can be an available goal to any individual in respect of the particulars of his or her health if he or she is in a fit and proper condition to participate fully in all the practical exercises in this book.

5. The Goal must be Located Within the Individual's Environment

The goal must be within your own environment or situation. For example if a person's goal is to be Prime Minister it follows that in order to achieve the goal, he or she must be a politician or else he or she never gets to achieve such a goal in a democratic country. What happens in countries which are not democratic, where anyone can buy their way into high office or just seize power by armed means, is exceptional rather than the norm.

As in our illustration above, to be Prime Minister of a democratic nation like the United Kingdom, for instance, a person must be in politics and win his or her seat in a general election. He or she must also be the leader of the party that won the general election or be the winner of a party leadership contest by challenging the incumbent Prime Minister directly, or the winner of a leadership election in the event of a resignation or death of a Prime Minister.

What is relevant from these illustrations is that being a politician in a democratic country places the individual in a situation from which he or she can fulfil a goal of being Prime Minister. However a British politician whose goal is to be the President of the USA would be setting his or her goal far beyond his or her environment and thus making it too difficult or relatively impossible to fulfil.

We would say from the above illustrations that the goal to give up smoking is ordinarily within the environment of any individual since giving up smoking entails what one does to oneself. However, the method by which an individual chooses to do this might be stringent and thus, remote to the individual's metabolism.

The method that we advocate in this book is positive thoughts about one's goals and aspirations. It is mental and so it is within the environment of any individual who is able to use his or her mind profitably in positive thoughts.

6. The Goal must be kept constantly in Mind

Remember from what we said above about the unconscious mind that your ideas must be clearly imprinted and fully developed in your mind for them to work for you. When you have taken the time and mental energy to formulate your goal, define it clearly and make a plan of action, it becomes necessary that you must keep the goal constantly in your mind in order to fulfil it.

It is quite obvious that failure to keep the goal constantly in your mind may result in your forgetting it completely or replacing it with other desires on your scale of preference. In the method we advocate in this book, the goal to give up smoking is a goal of mental action so it is much more amenable to be kept in the mind.

HOW TO DEFINE YOUR GOAL

Your goal must be stated clearly and precisely. One needs to be very specific in defining a goal. This is very important so that the action plans for achieving the goal are specifically directed and the mind is clearly focused on a particular goal. Your knowledge of the functions of the unconscious mind which we discussed above will help you to understand the need to be clear and specific in your definition of the goal.

The ultimate aim here is to fulfil your desire by giving up smoking now and to do so easily, completely and effectively. Notice that the element of time is already entailed by our title, 'Stop Smoking Now!' Thus, you can define the goal in the following terms and this will also form part of your relaxation exercise. In this way the goal will be firmly established in your mind.

Your goal is to stop smoking now and to do so completely, easily, effectively and to remain a non-smoker from this moment onwards. Giving up smoking, completely, easily and effectively will fill you with pleasure and happiness. You will feel the sensation of pleasure as you begin to breathe clearly and have more strength, energy and stamina day by day in every way.

You will regard each clear breath that you take as a sign of the success of your action plan and you will be very happy knowing that with each and every passing day from this moment onwards you are concerned more and more for the general improvement of the health and integrity of your body.

You will be totally relaxed and completely in control from this moment onwards because you know that you will achieve success with your goal to stop smoking now! When you give up smoking completely, easily and effectively and continue to be relaxed everyday you will find that the feeling of total relaxation, the feeling of being in control, the feeling of peace of mind and general well-being will stay with you and become part of your everyday feelings from this moment onwards.

You will be confident, positive, and optimistic in your outlook and you will love yourself because of the success you are achieving with your goal. From this moment onwards as you continue to feel positive and happy, you will be able to show a positive attitude of love towards the people that matter in your life and you do this by giving up smoking now and stop forcing them to become passive smokers by smoking around them.

The above is the goal clearly defined. This must be stated clearly and distinctly so that the unconscious mind understands your intention in relation to your goal of giving up smoking (or for whatever purpose). If the above definition of your goal is chosen it indicates to the unconscious mind that you want to give up smoking completely, easily and effectively as we stated above. In this way the unconscious mind will help you to accomplish your goal easily and effortlessly.

GAINING ACCESS TO THE UNCONSCIOUS MIND THROUGH DEEP RELAXATION

Now that your goal is clearly defined, you must induce yourself into a state of deep relaxation in order to gain access to the unconscious mind. You must begin with the following procedure.

How to induce yourself into a state of Deep Relaxation

Settle down and make yourself comfortable on a chair, couch or on the floor. Now, breathe in deeply, long and slow, through your nose.

Hold your breath for a mental count of 5, 10 (or whatever number is suitable for you), exhale gently and allow the air to spread through your body as you R E L A X. Repeat this three or four times (or as many times as it is possible to loosen yourself up).

Now imagine yourself out in the open air. Make it a beautiful place and a beautiful day just as you would like it to be. You may choose to be on a sandy beach, in a park or even in your back garden. Wherever it is that you've chosen to be at this moment in your mind, make it a place which represents for you the very ultimate in peace, joy and total relaxation.

As you continue to relax this way from day to day you will find that you will feel very peaceful with each and every passing day. This feeling of peace and total relaxation will become a part of the way you feel from day to day, it will become an attitude of mind and body for you. You will be very profoundly relaxed in mind and body wherever you happen to be and whatever the situation or the circumstances in which you find yourself, you will be absolutely relaxed and in control come what may.

Relaxation will give you the peace of mind and the inner tranquillity which enables you to deal with the stress, the tensions, the worries and the anxieties of everyday life.

Now allow the feeling of relaxation to surge through every part of your body more and more. Begin from the top of your head and feel your scalp and your forehead relaxing, feel the muscles around your eyes relax, feel your cheeks and the muscles around your mouth relax, feel the whole of your face relax.

This feeling of relaxation begins now to spread down from your face to your neck and throat and from there it spreads across your shoulders and from your shoulders through your arms to the tips of your fingers with your wrists and your elbows very deeply relaxed. Concentrate now on your chest and your upper back and feel relaxation spreading from your chest to your abdomen and from your upper back to your lower back so the trunk of your body is very deeply relaxed.

Now feel your waist and your bottom relax. This feeling of relaxation spreads to your pelvis, then your thighs, and from your thighs all the way through your knees and your lower legs to the tips of your toes. Your entire body relaxes. Now feel relaxation surging through your body from the top of your head to the tips of your toes and from the tips of your toes to the top of your head.

As you continue to relax this way, you will find that the stress and the strain of the day will go out of your mind and out of your body. With increased relaxation you are able to let go your worries and your anxieties and allow the feeling of peace and inner calmness into your body and into your life.

You are now feeling a deep, profound relaxation in every part of your body, every fibre, every atom and every particle of your body. Your entire body is now deeply relaxed and serene. With this relaxation you should feel peaceful and comfortable and as you become totally relaxed and completely in control, you may experience either a tingling sensation spreading through your body, or a feeling of lightness, or weightlessness as if you are about to fly away on your own, or a combination of those feelings.

As you are now deeply relaxed your unconscious mind is ready to receive positive instructions for your present and future well-being, for your happiness and to enable you to stop smoking now, easily and effectively.

Note

As you are now deeply relaxed, your unconscious mind is now ready to receive positive instructions or mental prompts for your present and future well-being, for your happiness and to enable you to stop smoking now, steadily, easily and effectively. This note can also be incorporated in your relaxation technique as I have done it above thus allowing your goal of stop smoking now, easily and effectively to be imprinted on your unconscious mind and become easily achievable by you.

The effect of this will be lasting for you because as your goal is imprinted in your unconscious mind your motor activities will reflect it. In this way the actions which will lead to the fulfilment of your goal will become part of your everyday motor activities. Refer to our fundamental principles in chapter one.

Positive Instructions or Mental Prompts

When you have attained a deep level of relaxation you can then give yourself positive instructions in relation to your desired goal which you have previously defined. These instructions will, indeed, be a repetition of the essential details of your goal as we have defined it, above. We have defined a goal for stop smoking now above.

Now for further illustration, let us suppose that you have another goal which is to eliminate pain from your body. Let us make it more interesting and suppose, further, that it is the elimination of period pains, pain of arthritis or pain during childbirth. Let us settle for pain during childbirth. Male readers may concentrate on the pain of arthritis or any other pain they may have. We may begin as follows.

From this moment onwards when you use the word R E L A X, you will immediately feel as relaxed, comfortable, and serene as you are now. The word R E L A X will mean complete calm, peace, confidence and total tranquillity in your entire being. When the contractions begin during the birth of your baby the word R E L A X will turn the contractions to pleasurable sensations within your body and you will feel calm and confident.

You will be serene and anaesthetised to the contractions while enjoying happy, pleasurable, sensations in your body. These pleasurable sensations are a sign that your baby is about to arrive. The sign of the arrival of your baby fills you with great joy.

*As you are relaxed, you will be in total control throughout the birth because of your confidence and your knowledge that you have the **inner power to switch off** any unwanted sensation in your body. You will be full of joy, full of energy and vitality. The contractions will give you a feeling of joy. You will feel joy in the knowledge that* *your baby is about to arrive and the contractions are necessary for the arrival of your baby. You will feel pleasure as your baby enters the birth canal and each movement in your body gives you a pleasurable sensation in the knowledge that the waiting is all over and your baby is about to emerge.*

The feeling of calm and confidence, joy and happiness will continue for you well after the birth of your baby and you will be always relaxed and in control, calm, full of confidence and contentment, full of energy and vitality day by day in every way. The birth of your baby will be a satisfying, pleasurable experience. You will feel totally relaxed and confident and you will show great love and affection for your baby and exhibit a positive attitude of love towards all your dear ones.

Note

Notice that we have used some of the positive expressions that we used at the preparatory exercises in chapter one. This is for familiarity. Your mind is already familiar with these positive words and will react to them positively when you focus your mind clearly on your objective. In this particular exercise, if you cannot remember the essential details of your goal, use a summary that contains the gist of what you want to achieve. Always use positive expressions and avoid the use of negative terms at all times.

Always affirm the things that you want to achieve not their negation. Here is an example of a positive affirmation.

"During the birth of my baby I will feel a pleasurable sensation in my body and I will feel calm, confident, totally relaxed and absolutely in control."

In contrast to the example above, consider the following statement as an affirmation.

"During the birth of my baby I will not panic, and I will not feel any pain."

The above statement is an emphasis on what the individual will not do. The emphasis must always be on what the individual will do. It is, therefore, a negative and dangerous affirmation in so far as it is focused on panic and pain. These are feelings which the expectant mother does not want during the birth of her baby. You must always be on your guard against the temptation to make such dangerous affirmation.

Note that we have used the pain of childbirth here merely for the purpose of illustration. Remember that the gist of the mental prompts in our illustration can be applied to your goal to stop smoking now and to remain as a non-smoker always and be able to feel good, generally.

The above procedure is what you need for your goal to stop smoking now. However, we shall learn more techniques in the next chapter so that you have the option to choose the method that suits you best.

KEY POINT TO REMEMBER

- It is necessary to be deeply relaxed in mind and body for the purpose of bringing about the desired changes.

Now let us examine how everything we have said here about goals fits in with an individual's actual goal of giving up smoking.

PROBLEM: THE 60 CIGARETTES A DAY SMOKER

A disturbed man gave us the following information about himself and his problem.

I am 45 years old and I have been a smoker for 30 years. I smoke cigarettes, not pipe. I smoke first thing in the morning and I smoke in bed too. I smoke after I have had a meal and I smoke cigarettes whenever I have any drinks such as alcohol, coffee or tea. Whatever drink I have, I smoke with it by force of habit. But I do not really enjoy it because smoking leaves a bad taste in my mouth.

I smoke because I can't help it, I have got to smoke or I'll have nothing. I am addicted to smoking and I think I have an obsession with the thoughts of smoking. It is something I must do to keep me going. Sometimes I cough heavily when I smoke and I have recently noticed that I am now coughing constantly as I have bouts of coughing every day, but I notice this in other people too so I do not worry about the cough.

I feel stressed and stretched out from day to day and I have no strength or energy for anything. I am always tired. I have been insulted often by people who tell me that I reek of smoke and that I have bad breath and, although I do not notice these things, they have begun to bother me seriously and I really want to stop smoking now.

STOP SMOKING NOW! GOAL: TO STOP SMOKING NOW!

Remember that we are dealing with **mind power,** how you can use the thinking power of your mind to achieve your goals successfully or how those who are negatively inclined can prevent themselves from achieving a desired success by their pathetic negative thoughts.

If you have followed our discussions attentively you would be able to see quite easily, clearly, the power of the gentleman's negative thoughts. By using your mind solely for negative thoughts you would be eliminating yourself from the benefits of the opportunities around you and, thus, preventing yourself from achieving the success that you would, otherwise, have enjoyed, yet blaming your failure on other people!

In the case of the *60 Cigarettes a Day Smoker* his addiction to smoking tendencies and negative thinking were preventing him from giving up smoking and enjoying good health with strength and energy. It is obvious that he wants to give up because the insults of other people have begun to bother him. His problem is introduced to us as a *complaint*. This indicates that the current situation is an unwanted situation, perhaps it is an intolerable situation. However he postpones the attempt to take positive action to deal with the situation by saying that he cannot help it because smoking is something he must do to keep him going. He also tells us that he must smoke or he will have nothing.

Now in making those statements as his reasons for smoking, he makes out that smoking is necessary for his life and, unconsciously, plays the *self pity* card which, in this instance, is a defence mechanism against taking a positive action to look after his health by taking precautions against the poison of further smoking. This form of defence is known as *rationalisation.* It sounds good on the surface but deep down it prevents the individual from taking positive action on any particular uncomfortable or unwanted situation. The *60 Cigarettes a Day Smoker* takes his stated reason for smoking to be an affirmation of truth and so does nothing about it.

This is, indeed, his problem. He is affirming what he does not want, that is, affirming the negation of what he really wants. So he gets what he affirms because this is what has been imprinted on the unconscious mind. His negative thinking provides him with an excuse for not bothering to take care of his general health and wellbeing.

There is, therefore, a conflict which is what is making it difficult for him to see the actual problem and, then, give up smoking. The conflict is between his unexpressed wish to give up smoking because it is dangerous to his health and his expressed belief that he must continue to smoke because it is what keeps him going. He must resolve this conflict in order to stop smoking completely, easily and effortlessly. He must remember that *there is always a way out of any problem* through the positive use of the powers of the mind.

With the idea of positive thoughts in mind, let us now turn the *60 Cigarettes a Day Smoker's* desire to stop smoking now into a goal to stop smoking now with the incentive of regaining his strength, energy and stamina, become fit and healthy and free from embarrassing cough and see how a positive frame of mind will help him to fulfil his desire. This positive frame of mind will be implicated in his beliefs, attitudes, the way he channels his energy and it is best described in an *action plan.*

HOW TO MAKE AN ACTION PLAN FOR THE GOAL: TO STOP SMOKING NOW!

The fulfilment of any goal requires a positive frame of mind which is defined in an action plan. An *Action Plan* is a definite plan of action, activities or tasks which must be performed in order to accomplish the goal. It sets out the course of actions, sets out the various actions which are necessary for the fulfilment of the desired goal. For our stated goal on behalf of the *60 Cigarettes a Day Smoker,* the necessary actions and attitudes must include action to eliminate smoking odour and action to improve strength and energy. The action plan can be stated as follows.

Action 1: Expressing Self Belief

- I can give up smoking completely, easily and effectively because I believe that I have the power to do so.
- I can give up smoking completely, easily and effectively because that is my goal.
- I can give up smoking completely, easily and effectively because I am concerned for my health.
- I believe that I am a very determined man who sets goals and fulfils them.

- I believe that I can be a non-smoker because that is what I want.
- I am a sociable person and I believe that smoking is now an anti-social behaviour.
- I firmly believe that the Hollywood image of smoking is now out of date. I will stop smoking now because I am a modern man who is a health conscious person.
- I know what I want and how to get it.
- I am a sociable man and a non-smoker

Action 2: Act with Positive belief and Show this in Attitudes about Smoking

- I believe that smoking is no longer a desirable habit.
- I will stop smoking now because I care about my health.
- I take particular care about my appearance because I like to feel good and look good always.
- I will accomplish my goal by my decision and determination to stop smoking now!
- I accept that smoking is dangerous to my health and I have given up smoking because I am concerned to regain and improve my strength which has been weakened and my energy which has been dissipated by smoking.

Action 3: Translating Action 2 into Positive Practical Action

- I care very much about eliminating odour from my clothes and my body
- I will always pay attention to my clothes and my personal hygiene.
- I will always pay attention to my overall appearance
- I will give up smoking completely and I will do so easily and effortlessly.

- I will refrain more and more from the habit of binge drinking of beer and wine.
- I will pay more attention to my overall physical appearance by doing exercises.
- I will practise the relaxation exercises outlined in this book.
- I will perform positive actions to give up smoking completely, easily and effectively.

Action 4: Be Confident in the Knowledge that You Are now a non-smoker

- Knowing something entails knowing that one knows it. The worth of knowledge is in its usage. The *60 Cigarettes a Day Smoker* must make use of his newly acquired knowledge and show constantly that he is now a genuine non-smoker. He must accept himself as a non-smoker and, henceforth, regard smoking as a bad habit which is an anti-social habit.
- The *60 Cigarettes a day Smoker* must affirm the knowledge and belief which is expressed in action plans 1 and 2 by showing confidence in his ability to stop smoking now!
- The *60 Cigarettes a Day Smoker* must be positive about his decision and determination to stop smoking by making certain that this is reflected in his social behaviour and health concerns.
- The *60 Cigarettes a Day Smoker* must endeavour to make use of the knowledge that he is now a non-smoker and make the commitment to remain a non-smoker from this moment onwards.
- The *60 Cigarettes a day Smoker* must perform all the activities which are amenable to the fulfilment of the goal to stop smoking now.

Action 5: Affirming the Goal

- The *60 Cigarettes a Day Smoker* must keep the goal constantly in his mind through a general positive outlook on the possibility of its attainment
- The *60 Cigarettes a day Smoker* must **go for it** and stop smoking now completely, easily, effectively and effortlessly in order to avoid the threat of bronchitis and emphysema, to feel good, look good and stop coughing.
- The *60 Cigarettes a Day Smoker* must affirm all the critical health and social reasons that were necessary for his journey to the world of positive possibilities (see chapter one). He must make that journey as often as necessary to maintain his non-smoker status.
- The general rule is for the *60 Cigarettes a Day Smoker* to remember his self worth and think of himself as a very sociable man who is a non-smoker (see action 1).

In the name of honesty, sincerity and his concern for his health, the *60 Cigarettes a Day Smoker* must make a firm decision about his concern for his health if he is genuine and serious enough to give up smoking. He must deal with conflict mentioned above by following the action plan rigidly in order to achieve the desired objective.

Notice that we have set the goal with a time element, *'Now!'* This time element is also part of the title of this book. It underlines both the urgency of the task in hand and the desire to give up smoking. It is the time element that transforms the *60 Cigarettes a Day Smoker's* desire to stop smoking now into a goal to stop smoking in order to look good and feel fit and healthy again. The time element fixes the goal on his unconscious mind. The actions necessary to accomplish this have an additional effect of helping the smoker to give up smoking. The time element helps the smoker to be serious about the actions necessary to accomplish the goal and enables the smoker to keep the goal constantly in mind.

Notice also that the goal and the plans for its achievement involve the *60 Cigarettes a Day Smoker* in new activities and in positive thoughts which bring about positive feelings. We have used a gentleman's complaint for our illustration. Depending on the context of a particular problem, the same procedures are also applicable for a woman.

HOW TO ACQUIRE THE WILL TO SUCCEED IN GIVING UP SMOKING

Remember that you must keep the goal alive in order to fulfil it. Refer to our fundamental principles in chapter one and you will find that the more deeply you understand the importance of the above factors, the more effectively you will be able to apply them in your daily life and so you will be successful in whatever undertaking you embark on and you will certainly be successful in giving up smoking completely, easily, effectively and effortlessly. If you put your mind seriously into achieving success in giving up smoking completely, easily and effectively you must go for it so that you stop smoking now!

Use your mind positively. Give up all restrictive negative attitudes and propel yourself to success because it is clear that out of the world of any endeavour, success begins with a fellows will to succeed. In every endeavour that you embark on, negative thoughts are the things that are most likely to prevent you from achieving the success that you desire.

Most important of all, you must always bear in mind the fundamental principles of mind power which we have discussed in the first section of this book. Remember that the thought bricks for success or failure are constructed in the mind and always endeavour to construct the bricks for success. Try to understand and master the following little verse which clearly underlines the fundamental principles of mind power which we discussed in chapter one of this book.

If you think you are beaten, you are.
If you think you dare not, you don't.
If you like to win, but think you can't,
It is a cinch you won't win.

If you think you will lose, you have lost.
For out of the world we find,
Success begins with a fellows will,
It is all in the state of mind.
If you think you are outclassed, you are.
You've got to think high to rise,

You've got to be sure of yourself before
You can ever win a prize.
Life's battles don't always go
To the stronger or faster man,
But soon or late the man who wins
Is the man who thinks he can.

(Anonymous)

In any particular situation, if you think you can, you are already on your way to the winning post. It is all in the state of the mind. Your success begins with your construction of effective thought bricks which entails the plan of action which you have made to attain the success which you need, this is the essence of mind power. Thus you must always attune your mind to success and you will be for ever successful.

Remember that *the magic of success is within you.* It is within your mind. Apply the magic now in everything that you do from day to day starting from today and you will find that you can stop smoking now! You can do so completely, easily and effectively by adhering to all the principles in this book.

CHAPTER THREE

Giving Up Smoking Completely, Easily and Effectively

If you have built castles in the air, your work need not be lost: that is where they should be. Now put the foundations under them (Henry David Thoreau, 1817—1867).

DEEP RELAXATION AS WEAPON FOR GIVING UP SMOKING

We have discussed deep relaxation for the goal of giving up smoking in the last chapter. In this chapter we offer other ways of arriving at deep relaxation for the same purpose. Now you have a choice of what methods to adopt. The procedure, that is the outline of what to do, is the same but the scripts, imagery and pictorial representation are different.

Always remember that deep relaxation is an indispensable aid to giving up smoking through our practical mind technique as it helps the individual to stay focused on the chosen objectives. In order to give up smoking completely, easily and effectively one must, first, learn how to attain a profound level of relaxation both mentally and physically. With practice, you will be able to attain your own required level of deep relaxation within minutes or seconds of your trying. It is that simple and we are going to try it right now. As the saying goes, *the taste of the pudding is in the eating.*

Surprisingly enough, most things within the field of depth psychology bear truth to the above saying. We are able to understand the techniques in the practice of depth psychology much better after we have been through it via therapeutic analysis for self knowledge in the nature of finding out more about our inner self. In like manner, in our particular case of giving up smoking, we are able to focus much deeper on our chosen objective when we are deeply relaxed or when we have developed a relaxed attitude as a way of life.

We are dealing with very practical personal affairs and the best method of approach in the application of practical matters is to practise by using the method you want to understand or learn about. With depth psychology one does not need to be ill or emotionally unbalanced in order to learn to understand one's inner self. Before the experience of self knowledge some people are usually ignorant objectors and a few may be uncritical apologists.

PRACTICE SESSIONS

In order to practice how to focus the mind to the idea of giving up smoking completely, easily and effectively, we proceed with a method of deep relaxation as follows.

1. Breathing Exercise

Firstly, find a comfortable position either sitting on a chair or lying on a couch or on a bed, or on the floor if that is more comfortable for you. Now take a long, slow deep breath through your nose. Hold your breath for a mental count of about 10, 20, 30, etc as desired. Choose the length of hold to suit your desired level of relaxation.

Then gently open your mouth slightly and slowly exhale as you allow the air out of your body and let go all negative thoughts as the air leaves your body and let go, let go, let go, let go, let go as you drift deeper, deeper and deeper, into peace, allowing the feeling of relaxation to spread from the top of your head all the way down to your toes. Repeat the process three times.

This means that you will be performing four breathing exercises in all. If you have done this properly, as you read these lines, you should feel the sensation of relaxation moving through your body, now. Your body should now feel all loosened up.

However, if you don't feel loosened up at this stage it is because you are tense, nervous or fighting with yourself in being sceptical, doubting your own ability to do it well. If this is the case, don't worry. I tell you that you can do it; it is really very simple. Now let go your negative thoughts and negative feelings and repeat the procedure until you feel loosened up. Start now.

There is no fixed rule on how many times you have to repeat the procedure. Many people feel at ease after one deep breathing exercise and some other people need to repeat the exercise a few times in order to feel at ease. Do what suits you the best, but do the exercise. Do not skip it over because it is a necessary part of the practice of giving up smoking with our practical mind technique.

Remember our fundamental principle above and try to think more about the great power of your mind and your ability to succeed in what you aim to achieve. If you truly believe that you can do it, you will. Always read the verse at the end of chapter two to encourage you and give you a confidence boost. However, if you feel any discomfort while doing the exercises, you must discontinue immediately and wait until you feel comfortable enough to continue.

2. Deep Relaxation Exercise

When you have completed the breathing exercises, your next move is to relax every part of your body by focusing your thought or concentrating your attention on each particular part of your body that you wish to relax.

When you have mastered this technique of deep relaxation, you will find that at any time you direct your thoughts to any part of your body and say to that part (or command it) to **r e l a x,** it will immediately obey your command. It will begin to relax and you will start to feel at ease straight away. This may sound implausible to you at first but with practice you will be able to prove it for yourself. When this happens you will be in control at any moment of tension or crisis.

In practising the techniques for giving up smoking, you will be speaking directly to your unconscious mind. Since we have already discussed the power of the unconscious mind and how it records the data of your life, you can now see how you can give up smoking easily, completely and effectively by recording your goals about giving up smoking directly in your unconscious mind as we did in the last chapter.

This is part of the mental programming which I mentioned above, you will be programming your mind to do what you want, in this case, to effect deep relaxation in your life. In this way you will be able to relax easily but, overall, the action plans for your goal will be manifested in your motor activity as you begin to perform, easily, effortlessly, all the everyday actions that are necessary to make your desire to give up smoking become a reality for you.

Note that it is much more effective to speak directly to your unconscious mind in the second person. However you may speak in the first person if you prefer. This is effective too. If this is what you want, you can adapt the text here to speak in the first person. You can now begin to speak to your unconscious mind by telling it to effect deep relaxation in your body. You may begin in the following way.

You are now entering a state of deep relaxation. Your feet are becoming more and more deeply relaxed. This feeling of relaxation is spreading upwards from the tips of your toes through your feet to your ankles, legs, knees and thighs. Your limbs are getting more and more relaxed.

The feeling of relaxation increases from your thighs and spreads to your bottom, your waist and your pelvis. This feeling of deep relaxation is slowly spreading to your abdomen, your stomach, your chest, and your back. You are getting more and more progressively relaxed. Your entire body is becoming relaxed and you feel very light and absolutely serene with relaxation.

Now, shift your attention to your hands as this feeling of serenity is spreading to all parts of your body. Your hands are becoming very deeply relaxed. The feeling of serenity and deep relaxation continues to flow upwards through your body from the tips of your fingers through your wrists, your hands, your elbows, your arms, all the way up to your shoulders.

Now as you are feeling relaxed, this feeling of relaxation surges across your shoulders so that your shoulders are deeply relaxed, very deeply relaxed. You now feel peace and tranquillity flowing through your whole body from all directions.

The feeling of relaxation continues to surge from your shoulders upwards to your neck and throat, and then across your face and up to the top of your head. Your scalp, your forehead, your cheeks, and your jaw are all very deeply relaxed. You are now experiencing a very profound feeling of relaxation in every part, every tissue, every atom, very organ, every consciousness and every system of your entire body.

The whole of your body is deeply relaxed, peaceful and comfortable. Your mind is calm, very quiet and tranquil. You are now perfectly in tune to give further information about giving up smoking to your unconscious mind. The information which you give will become part of your motor activity from now onwards and help you to give up smoking easily, completely and effectively.

Note that steps 1 and 2 above are known as *Induction*. In our discussion in the previous chapter, we have described this as *inducing yourself into a state of Deep Relaxation*. It is the same procedure but different way of arriving at deep relaxation. Do what suits you best.

3. The Instruction

You have now arrived at the crucial point at which to give dynamic instructions or mental prompts to your unconscious mind in order for your unconscious mind to produce the desired effect for you from now onwards. In the next section we shall deal with how to give this information to your unconscious mind.

Basically what we are saying is that when you have completed the breathing and the relaxation exercises correctly, you should be in the ideal frame of mind and disposition to programme your unconscious mind to effect the changes which you require in your life at any particular moment. In this instance we want to speak to the unconscious mind about giving up smoking easily, completely and effectively.

Always remember the fundamental principles we discussed in chapter one of this book. The thoughts that you have most often in your mind will become your reality. If the unconscious mind is fed constantly with your determination to give up smoking, this will become your reality and you will give up smoking easily, completely, effortlessly and smoking will cease to feature in your consciousness because you will eliminate its effect by eliminating it from your life permanently. You have done so easily, naturally, effortlessly because your unconscious mind has got the message.

It is that simple but we have to be serious about it for this to happen. We have to be specific about our intentions and speak to the unconscious mind in unambiguous terms. Remember that the unconscious mind reproduces things exactly as you have presented them, just like a tape recorder. It is also important that you believe, wholly and firmly, in what you are saying to the unconscious mind and not merely verbalise it parrot fashion.

THE DYNAMICS OF MENTAL PROMPTS

Mental prompts are personal instructions or personal information which you give to your mind with the desire for the particular instruction or information to become your reality. Our practical mind technique gives you the simplest method of recording information in the unconscious mind.

Remember that anything recorded in this way remains in the depth of unconsciousness but it is at the same time very active as it affects an individual's motor actions. Everything that we say to the unconscious mind in a deep state of relaxation remains in the unconscious but is manifested in our everyday motor actions. If you have forgotten about this you may now refer to our description of the power of the unconscious mind in chapter one.

Since your particular aim at the moment is to give up smoking easily, completely and effectively, the information which you give to the unconscious mind will reflect this aim in order to make your desired status of non-smoker a reality. This method of recording information in the unconscious consists of personal instructions given by you to your unconscious mind thus facilitating instant replay of the required information in your everyday motor actions.

We start in a simple way by giving simple information or instructions to the unconscious mind. Initially this will serve the purpose of getting yourself into the routine of giving mental prompts to the unconscious mind for the things which you desire to surface in your life through your everyday actions.

As you become adept in the use of mental prompts, you will find that the sky is the limit for you, because you can use the prompts to achieve anything you wish to achieve, to deal with anything in which you seek to achieve success. Indeed, to get what you want.

As you become relaxed and focus your mind deeply on what you wish to achieve, you will speak to your unconscious mind seriously about what you want to achieve. Soon with your actions, you will find that what you desire becomes your reality. Deep relaxation is the key to the success of mental prompts.

The personal instruction, or personal information, which we call mental prompts are mental directives ordering your unconscious mind to act on the information or instruction which you have given. Your unconscious mind acts on it to make your desire a reality. It works through your motor activities because, as we mentioned in chapter one and variously above, your unconscious mind acts on any information it receives.

Thus the personal instructions, or personal information which you give to your unconscious mind must be direct, definite, simple and, preferably, given mentally. However, you may give your orders or instructions audibly if this is more convenient for you. In whatever form you may wish to give your mental prompts, you must take note that it must be given during the moment of ultimate deep relaxation as mentioned above.

At this point of deepest relaxation you have established the optimum conditions to give your mental prompts of personal instructions or personal information for your unconscious mind to receive them freely. This point of ultimate deep relaxation is the moment at which your mind is absolutely receptive. You can see from this why it is more advisable to give the personal instructions or personal information mentally.

Whatever it is that you wish to accomplish in your life you can do so with our practical mind technique. To use the technique you will always make use of mental prompts but as we have mentioned above, it is always best to use the mental prompts technique of personal information or personal instruction immediately during the moment of ultimate deep relaxation.

If you have a lot of different instructions or information to give to your mind, you will find that it is very beneficial to put these in a sequence that is logical and meaningful to you. Remember that your unconscious mind is uncritical. It does not change what you say, it merely reproduces what you say, faithfully, to you. Thus, you must take particular care in the knowledge that your unconscious mind accepts information as presented. If what you say is careless, meaningless or ambiguous, your desired reality will not materialise!

It is also important that your mental prompts which consist of the personal instructions or personal information that you give to your unconscious mind should be in your own words, words that, as mentioned above, are meaningful to you and tailored to each specific area, problem or situation in your life which you wish to confront. Do not be rigid about this. Do whatever suits your particular requirements and what works best for you.

Give your instructions or personal information and, then relax and allow the unconscious mind to work on your instructions in order to make the instructions effective for you. For example, after you have used the relaxation technique and you feel that you are in the moment of ultimate deep relaxation, you may let your first personal instruction be to direct your unconscious mind to accept the word *r e l a x* as your instant cue for deep relaxation. You may begin to give this direction as follows.

From this moment onwards wherever you happen to be, whatever the occasion, whatever the circumstances, whomever you happen to be with, when you use the word 'r e l a x', you will become deeply relaxed immediately, comfortable and serene as you are now. The word 'r e l a x' will mean complete calm, peace and total deep relaxation in your entire being.

This is an excellent positive instruction at this stage because by it you are instructing your unconscious mind to make the feeling of deep relaxation a part of your life. What will happen with this mental prompt is that the feeling of deep relaxation will become an attitude of mind and body for you and you will cease to feel tense, edgy, nervous or irritable. You will be relaxed in difficult situations, come what may you will be in control, calm, relaxed in mind and body.

Notice that in the above instruction we said that *"you will become deeply relaxed immediately, comfortable and serene as you are now."* This is because the instructions should be given at the moment in your relaxation exercise when you attain a state of ultimate deep relaxation and feel peaceful and serene.

The purpose of the instruction, therefore, is to allow your unconscious mind to save this moment for you and make it a permanent part of your life which you can playback or bring on at any time you use the word *r e l a x*. Remember this, always. This is why you can order it and receive it because it is already there for you.

This act of giving simple instruction to your unconscious mind will bring about positive results in your life in whatever goal you wish to accomplish. It is important to distinguish the act of ordering, commanding or giving instructions to your mind from the act of giving suggestions. The act of ordering, commanding or giving instructions to your unconscious mind involves you in making a positive demand from your unconscious mind, ordering it to do what you want. It is like placing an order for something. Remember also the powerful force of the positive instructions in our preparatory exercise at the beginning of chapter one.

In the above example, you are giving an order which is to be executed by your unconscious mind to the extent that each time you use the word *r e l a x,* you will feel, from that moment onwards, an automatic and instant deep relaxation in mind and body. It will also bring about a highly desirable state of total calm whenever you desire it and wherever you happen to be, whether you are travelling on a crowded train, taking an examination, having a job interview, in a business meeting, participating in competitive sports event, driving a car in a busy traffic or in moments of minor personal crisis. All you need to do in these situations is say the word *r e l a x* and you will feel deeply relaxed, instantly.

The same procedure applies in giving up smoking. Remember that you have to be specific when making mental prompts. You must be clear and specific about the fact that you wish to give up smoking easily, completely and effectively. This is what you will ask for in your universal mental prompt or mind order. You want to eliminate smoking from your consciousness and become a non-smoker. This is what you will ask for or order for in your mental prompts.

FURTHER EXERCISES FOR GIVING UP SMOKING

Here we present relaxation exercises which will help you to give up smoking easily, completely, effectively and effortlessly. You do not need to try all of them although you may go through them and settle on the one that makes you feel comfortable. Remember that each of the exercises for giving up smoking begins with a method for deep relaxation. Follow the procedure which is given above. This procedure is incorporated in the exercises given below.

Using the Deep Relaxation as a method for Induction

Close your eyes and feel yourself relaxing gently as you keep your eyes firmly closed. Now imagine or picture, if you can, a scene of peace and tranquillity like the gushing of waves on a sandy shore, leaves rustling in a gentle breeze or whatever scene represents peace and tranquillity to you. Remember that the thoughts, pictures and images you have in your mind constantly are the things that will materialise into reality for you as these are charged with energy.

Now take a long, slow, deep breath through your nose. Hold the breath to a count of 5, 10 or whatever number that is appropriate for you. Now open your mouth gently and breathe out slowly as you relax, relax, relax. Feel yourself going deeper, deeper, and deeper into relaxation, becoming more and more progressively relaxed.

Now take a second long, slow deep breath through your nose. Hold the breath to a count of 5, 10 or the number that is appropriate to you, as before. Open your mouth gently and breathe out slowly as you let the air out of your body and relax, relax, relax, deeper and deeper.

Now take a third long, slow, deep breath through your nose and hold to a count of 5, or 10 as you wish as before. Now open your mouth and this time as you let the air out of your body gently, I want you to count the numbers from 10 to zero and relax as you go deeper, deeper, deeper and deeper into relaxation.

Using the Vibrant Energy of the Sun to Bring Peace and Serenity

Since we are appealing to the benefits of the *vibrant* energy of the light of the sun, it is best to use this exercise during the day time. If you have an urgent need to use it during the night time, you must modify the text to suit your purpose.

Now that you have completed the breathing exercise we will use the vibrant energy of the light of the sun to relax every part of your body. The light of the sun can be your instant cue to deep relaxation so that whenever you reach out, mentally, and bring it over to your body you will be deeply relaxed instantly. The light of the sun is, truly, your light in the dark, it helps you to see your way clearly wherever you are going and it signposts the directions for you, it guides you in whatever you are doing. The light of the sun is a positive light that helps you to achieve positive results in your life.

Now I want you to imagine that you find yourself out in the open air on a beautiful day. At this particular moment, you can choose to be in a park on a beach or on a holiday. The important thing is that wherever it is that you have chosen to be in your mind is a place which represents for you the very ultimate in peace, joy and total relaxation.

Imagine that the light of the sun is a healing light, a positive light, a light that represents joy, happiness, total fulfilment and every positive thing which you wish to feature in your life. The successful achievement of your goal is represented by the warmth of the healing rays of the light of the sun around you.

The light of the sun symbolises your success, your joy, your happiness and your achievement of your goal to give up smoking and fulfil your wish. Whenever you bring the light of the sun into your life you feel good instantly because it energises you, it dissolves your negative thoughts, worries and your anxieties. The light of the sun is a magical light because it brings success to you instantly, effortlessly. The light of the sun is your cue to instant deep relaxation in mind and body. Whenever you bring the light of the sun over to your body, you will feel deeply relaxed, instantly.

It is a beautiful day today. The light from the sun is warm and shining down through your body and it makes you feel good, positive and deeply relaxed. Stay with that feeling. Notice that the sky is an incredibly beautiful blue and there is a comforting breeze blowing across your body. You feel peaceful and deeply relaxed.

Now, I want you to reach up and bring the light of the sun to your body, bring it over to your right arm and focus it there like the ray or beam of a torch light and move it from the tips of your fingers all the way up to your shoulders. Move it backwards and forward, up and down until you can actually feel it in your mind the warmth of the light of the sun penetrating your skin, your muscles, your nerves and the bones in your body. You can feel your entire body beginning to relax more and more, deeper and deeper, becoming more deeply relaxed every minute.

Now move the light of the sun from your right arm to your left arm and from the tips of your fingers to your shoulders. Move it backwards and forward and imagine your left arm going deeply relaxed as your entire body settles down into deep relaxation as your sense and feeling of peace and tranquillity increases.

Bring the light of the sun over to your right leg and move it from the tips of your toes all the way up to your hip. As you breathe gently, you can actually feel your muscles relaxing and the tensions, the worries and the cares of the day just melting away out of your body and out of your mind. Your right leg and your toes all the way to your hip go deeply relaxed, very deeply relaxed.

Now move the light of the sun from your right leg to your left leg and from your toes to your hip and feel your left leg relaxing deeper and deeper and deeper. Now with both of your legs very, very deeply relaxed and both of your arms very deeply relaxed, you are using your own breathing as a guide and you can feel your entire body going deeper and deeper into relaxation with each breath that you take, with each thought and feeling and with each moment you are increasingly deeply relaxed.

I want you to know that some people feel light and weightless when they are deeply relaxed. They feel as weightless as if they could just float away. Other people experience a tingling sensation all over their body when they are deeply relaxed while some others have a feeling of elation or a feeling of peace and contentment. Whatever feeling you have at this moment should be a positive feeling and this is right and proper for you. Stay with your positive feeling and allow your mind to settle down as you go deeper, deeper and deeper into relaxation.

Gently now, bring the light from the sun into your stomach and feel it beginning to warm and to glow there. Feel it glowing like a ball of vibrant energy and feel the energy in every organ in your body. You can respond positively to this healing energy from the light of the sun as every organ in your body relaxes and you feel peaceful. You can feel the new found peace and tranquillity in your life as each day brings joy and contentment to you and your mind is filled with new and positive things to do which in their turn, make you feel peaceful, confident and optimistic about yourself and about the future. Stay with your peaceful feeling as you go deeper, deeper and deeper into relaxation.

Now, as you move the light of the sun into your heart through your chest you can actually experience, feel and know what it feels like to take this healing energy of the sun into your body, into your blood stream. Feel it moving out into every organ in your body and every organ is responding, healing and relaxing. Notice that your mind is becoming very peaceful and you have a feeling of joy and happiness. This is how things should be for you from now onwards.

Now, I want you to shift your attention to your back. Bring the light of the sun to your back and move it gently up and down your back. Move it across your back. Feel it massaging your back as the feeling of relaxation spreads from your upper back to your lower back and across your waist as the whole of your back goes deeply relaxed, very deeply relaxed.

Now as you bring the light of the sun into your body through your head you notice that the light moves to your spine. Notice that when the light gets to your spine, it begins to move out to all areas of your body. From your spine the light begins to radiate to every part of your body and every part of your body is relaxing accordingly.

Feel it now, the healing light of the sun is radiating to every organ in your body and every organ in your body is becoming active, alive and relaxing deeply. Every organ in your body is becoming healed by the light of the sun and every organ is now working well as it should. Relax and allow the healing process to begin in your body, allow the positive changes to takes place in your body and in your life from now onwards.

Now as the light from the sun moves across your shoulders, the burdens, the cares, the worries and the anxieties of the day just fall away from your shoulders and you are at ease. Notice that your forehead relaxes, your scalp relaxes, your neck relaxes, the muscles around your eyes and cheeks relax. Allow every part of your face to relax freely and allow yourself to go into a deeper, more blissful, more comfortable state of relaxation.

You are now relaxed, very deeply relaxed. You are at ease with what is happening now in your mind and body and very much at peace with what is being made available to you now.

In a few moments time you will be giving mental prompts to your unconscious mind asking it to receive certain information or instructions from you and to act on it as part of your everyday motor activities. These mental prompts will act to strengthen your determination to give up smoking, your desire, your will power and your self control. The mental prompts will fortify you in mind and body and will make it possible for you to maintain your integrity and your goal to give up smoking. Each and every mental prompt will have a unique effect upon you.

The mental prompts will grow stronger and stronger in you and become more and more effective for you from this moment onwards. The mental prompts will become totally a complete part of your everyday motor behaviour, totally and completely effective for you immediately. You can also add to their strength and effectiveness because each and every time you have a longing or a great desire to smoke you will be automatically reminded to count the numbers down mentally from ten to zero and, as you do this, you will notice that your longing or desire to smoke is easily eliminated.

Each and every time you do this you will find that the mental prompts have a unique effect on you. Remember the principle that the ideas which you have most often in your mind will become your reality. Remember the power of the unconscious mind.

You are now very deeply relaxed, very, very deeply relaxed. You feel a definite sense of peace moving over your body. Now imagine yourself back on that beautiful place in the open air where you were a moment ago. Be there at the count of five to zero. Five, four, three, two, one, zero. You are there.

Notice that the light from the sun is warm and shining down around your body and you have a feeling of peace, tranquillity and total relaxation. As you continue to relax in this way you will find that through the days and nights from now onwards, with your increased deep relaxation, the thoughts and desires of smoking have been eliminated easily and effortlessly.

Each and every mental prompt given here will be a permanent part of you for your mind is being programmed now to receive the mental prompts and you will act on them automatically, involuntarily, unconsciously. You will begin carrying out the dictates of the mental prompts in your motor activities and they will become effective for you immediately. These mental prompts will change your attitude to smoking because you now have much more self control, much more will power and much more determination to succeed in your desire to give up smoking than ever before.

I want you to stay relaxed and go deeper, deeper and deeper. I want you to realise from now onwards that with each and every passing day you have the power to obtain whatever you desire. The power to get whatever you desire is truly within you and your desire at this moment is so intense that you can actually visualize yourself becoming a non-smoker because that is what you desire. Remember your journey to the new world of positive possibilities. You can make that journey again at anytime you choose as it will help you to actualize your goals.

Cleaning and Purifying your Lungs

Now that you are deeply relaxed, I want you to come with me for a journey into the inside of your body. I want you to be there at a count of five to zero. Five, four, three, two, one, zero. You are now inside your own body. I want you to imagine that the inside of your body is now filled with a restorative antibacterial and antibiotic liquid detergent that is soothing and calming to your body. This liquid will clean, disinfect and purify your internal system. The liquid has two vital roles to fulfil for you in relation to your wish to give up smoking.

The first vital role of the liquid is that as a detergent, it will clean and purge all your desire and thoughts of smoking and wash these out of your mind and out of your internal system for good. The second vital role of the liquid is as antibacterial and antibiotic it will restore, heal, soothe and calm the nerves that have been severely damaged and ravaged by smoking. The liquid will wipe out the deposits of tar, nicotine and the poisons from your lungs and keep your lungs and your internal system fresh.

I want you to concentrate your attention now on your lungs. Listen to the cleaning work being down by the liquid. Feel it now, scrubbing, cleaning your lungs. Notice that there is still more work of cleaning to be done and I want you to step in and help out. So, I want you to imagine that you are a cleaner. Your job is to go into your lungs and clean it out thoroughly. I want you to be there at the count of five to zero. Five, four, three, two, one, zero. You are now a cleaner in your lungs.

Notice that your lungs are as dark as the inside of a chimney and there is a mass of wreckage, soot and rubbish left there by the effect of smoke. Your job is to clear the debris and to clean your lungs of the tar, the nicotine and the poisons that are left there by the impact of smoke. You can use whatever is necessary and you can use the liquid detergent to help you. I want you to begin now. Clean both sides of your lungs. Clean out all the filthy rubbish and use the liquid detergent to freshen the smells. Well done, you have done an excellent job.

Now your next job is to move from your lungs to your spine. I want you to be there at the count of five to zero. Five, four, three, two, one, zero. You are now in your spine. I want you to notice that many of the nerves of your body are connected to your spine and the nerves have been severely damaged and ravaged by the effects of smoking. Your job now is to take the sponge that is in the liquid detergent and use it to apply the liquid gently on your nerves from your spine all the way to your brain. I want you to notice that as you apply the liquid to your nerves, your nerves will become relaxed and the ravages and damage in them are healed. Continue to do this from your spine to your brain and I will join you at the centre of your brain in a hall where all the sockets and plugs with smoking are connected. Begin now to apply the liquid to your nerves to repair the damage caused by the effect of smoke.

Pulling out the Plugs and Sockets from Unnecessary Smoking Connections

You have applied the liquid to your nerves from your spine to your brain and you are now in a hall at the centre of your brain. Now, look around you and notice that the hall where you are is like an electrical power station with many plugs and sockets connected. These plugs, sockets and their connection represent your emotional, mental, physical and psychological association with the unwanted habit of smoking. Your job now is to disconnect the plugs and sockets. As you disconnect them, you will disconnect yourself now and permanently from the unwanted habit of smoking and you will stop smoking for good.

Now, whatever you smoke, there is a plug and socket there that represents your first smoke of the day. I want you now to reach out in your mind and discount the plug and socket which represent your first smoke of the day and you will stop smoking.

If you have associated smoking with a feeling of relaxation, I want you to pull out the plug and socket that represent this association, disconnect them now and you will stop smoking. It is important for you to know that you are very deeply relaxed now without smoking and you can be relaxed easily, completely, effectively and peacefully at any time you choose, without smoking.

If you have always smoked before, during or after a meal I want you to pull out the plug and socket that connect smoking with eating a meal and you will stop smoking. From now onwards you will enjoy perfect health with increased stamina and vitality because you are eating without smoking before, during or after the meal.

If you have associated smoking with being in control, being smart, being fashionable, being superior or being in authority you must now pull the socket and plug that connect smoking to these situations, positions and attitudes and stop smoking immediately for you can be all these things more effectively, without smoking.

If you have associated smoking with a fashionable, friendly and sociable activity which is performed on social occasions, you must pull out the socket and plug now and stop smoking for it is quite in order for you to be friendly, fashionable and sociable without smoking.

Some people turn to smoking as a solution to certain emotional problems in their lives or they may be insecure and turn to smoking for some superficial social reasons. If you have always turned to smoking as a solution to a feeling of anger, tension, nervousness, irritability, you must now pull out the socket and plug which represent your attempt to solve these emotional problems by smoking. You must stop smoking immediately because smoking creates and aggravates these emotional problems.

Some smokers use smoking as a form of oral gratification. They have an unfulfilled, unconscious, need to put something in their mouth as a substitute for what is lacking. If you have been using smoking as an oral gratification, you must pull out the socket and plug that links smoking as a substitute, oral gratification. Pull out the socket and plug now and you will stop smoking immediately.

Some people have been badly influenced into smoking by the Hollywood image of famous film stars smoking. These people feel that smoking will make them appear mature, attractive and sophisticated like the Hollywood stars that they idolize. Remember that the idea which is conjured by the image of the big stars of Hollywood smoking is now out of date and unfashionable. If you have been smoking because you think that smoking makes you look attractive, mature and sophisticated, you must pull out the socket and plug that represent these reasons for you and you will stop smoking and embrace a new way of living with care and concern for your health.

Other people smoke because of peer pressure, it is the only way that they can belong with the gang. If you have been smoking in order to become one of the gang, you must understand that this makes you insecure. So pull out the socket and plug that represent smoking with being a member of the gang and stop smoking now.

Now, I want you to notice that there is only one socket and plug left. This is the socket and plug that represent your last smoke of the day. I want you to pull out the last socket and plug which represent your last smoke of the day and disconnect yourself from smoking for ever and you will stop smoking immediately. Pull the socket and plug out now! Well done, you have done excellent work.

The cleansing of your internal system is now complete. The liquid detergent has done its job effectively and it is now time to allow what is left of it to flow out of your body. It will flow out of your body at the count of five to zero. Five, four, three, two, one, *zero. Allow the liquid detergent to flow out of your body now. As the liquid detergent flows out of your body, it carries with it the very thought of smoking itself, the nicotine, tar and poisons. As the liquid flows out of your body, you can see how filthy and repulsive it is, it is like sludge. As the liquid detergent now flows completely out of your body, I want you to have a look at your lungs now. Notice that your lungs now look clean and fresh and that you are now breathing clearer and easier.*

You are now deeply relaxed, very, very deeply relaxed. You have a feeling of peace and total relaxation moving all over your body. Now, I want you to imagine yourself back in that place in the open air, and make it a beautiful day. I want you to be there at a count of five to zero. Five, four, three, two, one, zero. You are there. I want you to notice that the light of the sun is warm and shining down around your body and the feeling is one of peace and contentment with the knowledge that you have now given up smoking and you have done so easily, effectively, effortlessly.

You will now receive powerful, positive, suggestions which will be very beneficial to you. Each suggestion will become part of your everyday motor response or motor behaviour. You will act on them automatically and they will become effective immediately because they are powerfully constructed to help you to stop smoking now!

From now onwards, you will think positive thoughts so that positive feelings will flow to you about your new status as a non-smoker. Whenever negative thoughts of smoking attempts to enter your mind and consciousness you must cancel them immediately by focusing your mind on your new status as a non-smoker, take a long, slow deep breath and count the numbers from 10, 9, 8, 7, 6, 5, 4, 3, 2, 1, zero.

You will notice that each time you cancel negative thoughts from your mind, take a long, slow, deep breath and count the numbers down from 10 to zero, you become more relaxed, positive and resolute as a non-smoker. With practice this will become more effective for you as the very thought of smoking will be eliminated from your life permanently.

You have now given up smoking. From now onwards you will become more and more relaxed with people, with members of your family and the people with whom you associate in daily life. Members of your family and your close associates will notice the change in your attitudes to smoking and how it has brought pleasant changes in you as a person and they will all be delighted for you and with what you have achieved. This will encourage you, even more, to give up smoking for ever.

From this moment onwards your impulse, desire, need, habit or urge for smoking has been terminated for ever. Smoking has now lost its hold on you as you now regard smoking as a sign of immaturity and insecurity.

You recognised that there is a great deal about smoking that is unpleasant so you made the great decision to stop smoking and, having stopped smoking, you will experience the most tremendous sense of accomplishment.

You are now a non-smoker and your determination, your self control, your will power and your self respect have all increased. You know now that smoking is a harmful and dangerous habit. You are now aware that smoking can lead to heart disease, lung cancer, emphysema and bronchitis. You are now aware of the amount of money involved in smoking and how you would love to use the money to do something beneficial for yourself or for the people around you. You are aware of the dangers of smoking to children, unborn babies and the people around you all of whom have been forced to become passive smokers by your selfish habit of smoking around them. You are now aware of the unhygienic effects of smoking such as the smell of smoke which you carry along with you, bad breath, ashes on your clothing, stained teeth and stained fingers.

When you consider these problems of smoking you made the wise decision to give up smoking immediately. From the moment that you stopped smoking you will begin to feel better during the day and you will begin to sleep more soundly, your health will improve and your mind will be clear and alert and you will feel better about life generally. You will have much more self control, determination and will power to resist the temptation to smoke. You will be able to resist the temptation to overeat and so you will maintain your ideal weight because your mind controls what you eat.

Now that you have stopped smoking and smoking is now in your past, you are very glad that it is now over, that you have given up the bad habit of smoking and you have done so easily and effortlessly. You have now developed a special feeling of superiority over the people who smoke because you know that they lack your self control, your determination, your will power, your sense of self worth and self respect. From now onwards, smoking will cease to feature in your consciousness. You have stopped smoking and you feel very good about yourself and your wise decision to stop smoking.

Now, I want you to take a long, slow deep breath and count the numbers down from ten to zero. You will be ten times more deeply relaxed and you will relax on each and every descending number. Every number down will be a step to peace and contentment and it will give you a feeling of accomplishment. Ten, nine, eight, seven, six, five, four, three, two, one, zero. Whenever you take a long, slow, deep breath and count the numbers down from ten to zero, your determination, will power and self control will be strengthened making it easy for you to maintain your resolution to stop smoking now! You will carry out all the positive suggestions that your unconscious mind has accepted and recorded faithfully for you and these will become effective in your life. These positive suggestions will become stronger for you and they will grow stronger day by day in every way and you will be happy that you have stopped for ever.

A Retrospective Journey

We are now going to move forward in time to allow you to look back in time and experience your self as a non-smoker who is thrilled by the joy and happiness of giving up smoking for ever. This journey forward in time is like your journey to the world of positive possibilities. At the end of the journey you will return to the world of actuality to actualize everything. Remember that if you can visualize it, you can also actualize it.

At the count of five to zero, I want you to imagine that it is now six months since you stopped smoking and you are feeling good about yourself. Five, four, three, two, one, zero. It is now six months since you stopped smoking and you are feeling good about yourself. So relax as you move forward and forward in time.

At the next count of five to zero, it will be one year since you stopped smoking and you will be feeling terrific about your wise decision to stop smoking and about the general improvement in your health since you stopped smoking. Five, four, three, two, one, zero. It is now one year since you stopped smoking and you are feeling terrific. So relax, as you move forward and forward in time.

At the next count of five to zero, it will be two years since you stopped smoking and you will be feeling happy that you have stopped the bad habit of smoking. The count now is five, four, three, two, one, zero, It is now two years since you stopped smoking and you are feeling quite happy about it. So relax, as you move forward and forward in time.

At the next count of five to zero, it will be three years since you stopped smoking and you will be feeling wonderful about yourself. Five, four, three, two, one, zero. It is now three years since you stopped smoking and you are feeling absolutely wonderful day by day in every way. So, relax and relish you sense and feeling of accomplishment.

You are relaxed, very, very deeply relaxed and you are happy knowing that you have made a positive decision to stop smoking and you have made the decision easily, firmly and correctly. Your mind is continuously in the moment of now and you take credit for your success with each and every passing day in the knowledge that you have stopped smoking for ever.

Now, I want you to bring the powerful light of the sun as a shield to protect you from the negative thoughts of smoking; bring it over to the top of your head to relax you and to cleanse you. Day by day in every way from now onwards, you will have much more energy and vitality as a result of your positive decision to effect changes in your life by giving up the bad habit of smoking. You will feel happy by this in the knowledge that you have stopped smoking for ever.

Now, as I count the numbers upwards from one to five, you will sit up at the count of five and your mind will become clear and you will feel refreshed and alert, healthier and feeling much better than you have ever felt before and you will be able to go about your normal activities and face your day (or night) with renewed strength, energy, joy, happiness and vitality with the knowledge that you have stopped smoking for ever.

1. *You can feel the healing energy of the light of the sun entering your body, making you feel alive.*
2. *You are feeling alert and happy with a smile forming on your face.*
3. *You are now feeling good and happy with the knowledge that you have now stopped smoking and you have done so easily, effectively and effortlessly.*
4. *There is a broad smile on your face, a warm, more comfortable feeling of accomplishment with the knowledge that from now onwards you will have more energy and vitality as a non-smoker.*
5. *The number 5 has been counted. You can open your eyes now and sit up with a clear knowledge that you have stopped smoking and you have done so easily and effortlessly. Well done. You are now a non-smoker.*

POSITIVE SUGGESTIONS FOR GIVING UP SMOKING

An Alternative Method

In this exercise, you can use any of the techniques for relaxation and induction as given in the exercises in the previous chapters.

Our chief aim in this exercise is to emphasise the positive aspect of being a non-smoker as we draw attention to the detriments of being a smoker. Basically this exercise is intended to make the smoker to become averse to the habit of smoking.

Now I want you to cast your mind back to your journey to the new world of positive possibilities. I want you to reflect for a moment on the health and social reasons which made the journey a necessary journey for you. As you reflect on this, you will find from now onwards that you will be more and more strongly aware of the reasons for giving up smoking and you will be more and more conscious of the threat to your health, of the increased chance of dying an ugly, painful, death from heart disease or cancer. You will be aware of the threat of fighting for each breath with bronchitis or emphysema or of causing sever damage to the arteries or veins in your body.

Many hardened smokers try to dismiss these threats and comfort themselves with the thought that it takes a long time to die from smoking. It is true that people do not die directly from smoking but each puff from smoking is a direct contributory cause of smoking related diseases whose threat become imminent as you continue to smoke.

Even now you will notice the way smoking interferes with your healthy life style, the gradual decline in your health, fitness and stamina, the shortness of breath which you get when you try to run, play other sports or climb stairs. There is also the bad breath that comes with smoking and the loss of the sense of smell and sense of taste.

You will ponder on the cost of smoking. Think about how much money you are spending on smoking from week to week, month to month or within one year. Work out this amount and think of how you could have used this amount to improve your health or to do something more beneficial to you.

From this moment onwards you will be more and more aware that smoking is becoming less and less acceptable in public and in social places. Smoking is now an anti-social behaviour in public places because it is dangerous to the people around you and you are, callously, forcing them to become passive smokers against their will.

Some people smoke because they think that smoking makes them feel big, relaxed and important but they know, deep down, that smoking makes them tense, nervous, snappy and irritable. Smoking is a nauseating habit. You will notice that if you continue to smoke from now onwards, you will be embarrassed and disgusted with yourself for being involved with such an anti-social and unhealthy habit and you will have an overwhelming unpleasant, sickening, feeling of nausea.

The unpleasant, dangerous, effects of smoking will take over in your mind and you will notice that you will no longer be able to smoke. When this happens you will know that your urge to smoke has disappeared and that smoking has lost its hold on you.

In addition to your realization of the unpleasant, dangerous effects of smoking, your unconscious mind knows all your reasons for wishing to stop smoking and it will find a safe way for you to stop smoking now because the reasons for your necessary journey to the new world of positive possibilities are imprinted on your unconscious mind. This can be played back to you each time you reflect on the journey to the world of positive possibilities. When this happens, you will be unable to smoke again for your desire to smoke will be dissolved by your unconscious mind and your craving for any particular method of smoking will disappear completely from your life. From that moment onwards, smoking will be very repugnant to you and you will develop a feeling of superiority over the people who smoke because you know that you have acquired a new social behaviour as a non-smoker and that smokers are anti-social.

From the moment that you stopped smoking, you will cease to notice and acknowledge smokers because the habit of smoking has been dissolved from your life and it has gone out of your consciousness. You will feel confident, positive and optimistic with the knowledge that you have stopped smoking for ever.

As your confidence grows with your new knowledge, you will become more and more proud of your self control, your self respect, your determination and your will power. You will feel healthier and look healthier, your will breathe well with your lungs, you will have more energy and your level of fitness and stamina will be greatly increased. You will feel good about yourself and about your life and your new life style as you discover that you can enjoy life more beneficially without smoking.

You will be calm and very much relaxed day by day in every way. As you are now a non-smoker, you will notice that you enjoy your food better as it tastes better because the bad taste in your mouth and the bad breath associated with smoking are now gone and out of your life. As you become more and more relaxed from day to day, you will begin to pay more attention to your health in general and you will be eating healthy food to remain healthy at all times. As a result of your new healthy regime and healthy eating habits, you will see that you will be able to enjoy your food and maintain your ideal weight when it is necessary to do so. You will, also, be able to protect your body from the dangerous effect of nicotine, tar and poisons which may come from the threat of further smoking.

As you continue to pay great attention to your health and enjoying healthy foods, you will feel stronger and stronger, healthier and healthier, from now onwards. In this way your resistance to smoking related illness and disease will increase and become stronger, steadily, day by day in every way. You know that for the sake of your health and social life, it makes very good sense to give up smoking. Your journey to the new world of positive possibilities has been beneficial to you enormously. It has helped you to realize the necessity to give up smoking and the ease with which you can do so. You have now given up smoking completely, easily and effectively. You have done so effortlessly with the power of your unconscious mind which records your positive intentions. Now you can count the numbers from one to five as in previous exercises in order to come out of deep relaxation. Well Done.

HOW TO MAKE THE HABIT OF NON-SMOKING YOUR REALITY

You can give up smoking easily, effectively and effortlessly because you have a firm desire to be a non-smoker. Your desire will become your reality soon. Remember that the thoughts which you have most often in your mind become your reality. If you can bring your thoughts into pictures and see them clearly then you can realise them easily and effortlessly. This is one way in which your dreams become your reality.

In this relaxation exercise, you will learn how to picture your desires and realise them. Remember also our journey to the world of positive possibilities in our preparatory exercise in chapter one. You can make the same journey now and try to see yourself as a non-smoker so that this will become your reality in the actual world.

In order to perform this exercise effectively, follow the steps as in our previous relaxation exercises and concentrate on seeing yourself as a non-smoker. Visualize yourself as you would like to be and use effective mental prompts at the moment of optimum relaxation.

GOING FOR YOUR SUCCESS IN GIVING UP SMOKING

Going For Success with Confidence

If you have followed everything that we have discussed here so far with attention then you have grasped the essential ingredients of the recipe for success in the use of your mind to get what you want. Always remember that whatever success you achieve in whatever field comes through your effective use of your mind to build an impregnable mind castle.

You must now consolidate on what you have gained from this book. To do this you must display confidence in yourself and in your ability to succeed in your chosen field, that is, in your ability to stop smoking now easily, completely and effortlessly.

You can display this confidence by translating the secrets you have found in this book, your new found pattern of belief system, your new wealth of ideas regarding the unpleasant and dangerous effects of smoking, your positive attitudes and positive frame of mind in respect to yourself and your goals and aspiration, etc, into action. Do not be afraid to achieve success, be resolute about your desire to achieve success in giving up smoking now. We have discussed various mind techniques for giving up smoking in this chapter and various methods of relaxation in this book.

Practise the method that you feel most comfortable with but you must practise because action is the essential ingredient that brings success in any goal. Now, you must take the bull by the horn with courage and boldness and you will be successful in your goal. Do not procrastinate for procrastination is negative thinking. I say to you, **go for it with confidence so that you can Stop Smoking Now!**

Believe me, you can be a great success in any venture if you think you can. You must think constructive thoughts supported by positive action. I mentioned the *Cogito* in the first chapter of this book to illustrate the power of thought. Now here is a new slant to the *Cogito*.

I think that I have the power within me to give up smoking easily, completely and effortlessly, therefore, I can stop smoking now!

Now think about that, articulate it by action, doing something new. Remember the principles of mind power, if you truly believe that you can do it then, so be it, you can. Remember that a true belief in our sense is one that is like faith and ignites serious positive action.

PRACTICE SESSIONS

How to Give Yourself A Confidence Booster

Follow the method which we have discussed above and proceed with personal instructions about what is to be done, then follow up with deep relaxation and finally the essential positive mental prompts at the moment of ultimate deep relaxation.

If you think that it is more convenient for you to listen to your positive mental prompts, then you may record them on a CD or on an audio tape if you have still got one of those and listen to your recording regularly. Your mind will absorb it quicker because you will be listening to your own voice, the ideas become your thought bricks and the effect of listening to them is astonishingly therapeutic. We give a guide here. The guide is as given before, the same order, different words, pictures and imagery so you have many to choose from each of the chapters of this book. You may proceed as follows.

Instructions

To begin with, find yourself a very comfortable position, sitting or lying down and proceed as follows. Put yourself into a state of deep relaxation in accordance with the methods which we have demonstrated in this book. While remaining in this deeply relaxed state, give yourself positive mental prompts for the idea of success in giving up smoking easily, completely and effectively as follows.

Relaxation

Take a long, slow, deep breath through your nose, not your mouth, hold it to a mental count of five. Now open your mouth slowly and gently exhale all the air from your body as you allow the feeling of relaxation to spread through your body from the top of your head to the tips of your toes. As you relax, you will think positive thoughts about success in giving up smoking easily, completely, effectively and effortlessly. Now go deeper, deeper and deeper into peace, going into a higher state of consciousness in relation to the idea of giving up smoking completely, feeling completely fresh from the inside, feeling good and looking good.

Positive Mental Prompts

From this moment onwards you will think positive thoughts so that positive feelings will flow to you in relation to success in giving up smoking, easily completely and effectively. You have let go your tense hold on negative thoughts and negative emotions and you have let go past disappointments in your attempts to give up smoking or in any area of your life. The past will cease to bother you from now because you have great confidence in yourself and in your plans for giving up smoking now! You have planned the way you want to live your life, your life will be free from smoking from now onwards and the future will be exactly what you want it to be, it will be according to your plans. You will give up smoking, easily, completely and effectively, you will be fit, healthy and energetic because you have given up smoking. You will look good and feel good from now onwards.

You have eliminated restrictive mental frameworks relating to the idea of success in giving up smoking easily, completely and effectively. You've let go mistaken beliefs relating to what you want to achieve so your success in giving up smoking will come to you through your positive thoughts and attitudes. Your mind is now clearly attuned to success in your chosen goal so your goal to give up smoking will be achieved easily, completely, effectively and effortlessly. You are genuinely and seriously concerned with success. You will achieve success because you are a determined person. You are firm and resolute in your search for success so you will derive great satisfaction from giving up smoking easily, completely, effectively and effortlessly.

Day by day in every way from now onwards, as you relax you will find that the road to success in your goal of giving up smoking is clearly sign-posted for you and you will get there and walk on the road of success, where you belong. You know that success in giving up smoking easily, completely and effectively is possible for you because everything is possible with the power of your mind.

Everyday in every way as you relax more and more, you will find that relaxation will give you the peace of mind and the inner tranquillity which will enable you to develop much more confidence in yourself and also much more confidence in your ability to do the things that matter in your life, the things that will bring greater success to you in giving up smoking easily, completely and effectively.

From this moment onwards you will be self-reliant. You are now full of independence and you have a determination to achieve success in your goal to stop smoking now. You have a great inner courage to succeed. Feel it now. Listen to your inner self. Everyday in every way from this moment onwards you will become more and more self confident as each day brings success to you in whatever you do from day to day.

You will begin now to project a new, positive, self image and you will be successful. As success begins to take over in your life, you will find that you will be happier and contented with what you are doing, much more cheerful and much more optimistic about your future in relation to your goal to stop smoking now. You will use your mind much more clearly and effectively as you come to appreciate the enormous power of your mind to bring success into your life. You will know it to be true that the magic of success is truly within you.

You can now make decisions easily, readily and correctly. As the decisions you make bring successes into your life with each and every passing day, you will find that your life is filled with rich and excitingly rewarding things to do to bring you further success, joy and happiness. So, go for it now with confidence and you will always be successful in anything you do as you give up smoking successfully easily, completely and effectively.

AFFIRMATIONS TO BRING THE RESULTS
THAT YOU DESIRE

Affirmations to help you to stop smoking now

Affirmations have truly magical powers which bring desired results to genuine seekers of success. We have been stating the general rule with affirmations all through this book.

The rule is that you must always affirm what you want to achieve, not the negation of what you want to achieve. You must not affirm the things, conditions or state of affairs which you do not require in your life. In brief you must always affirm your wishes, desires, intentions, goals, etc and not the negation of your desire or intention.

You must never deal with the negation of your intentions, just say what you want, not the negation of what you want. Let us give an illustration as follows.

I am a non-smoker.
I am a confident, positive and very optimistic person.
I am happy, cheerful and relaxed at all times.

The above statements are positive affirmations of the qualities and moods you wish to retain in your life. In contrast to the above, examine the following statement.

I do not want to be unhappy and I am not tense and not angry.

You must always guard against the temptation to make such statement as the one above because it is the affirmation of the negative traits which you should always avoid. The general rule is to concentrate on what you want and affirm it. In the above statement the emphasis is on *unhappy, tense* and *angry*. These are the traits you do not want but they are the ones that the unconscious mind has received so, unfortunately, those traits will underline your mood! If you are uncertain about this you can refer to our discussion on the unconscious mind in chapter one.

Affirmations are very powerful thought bricks of the mind. They work because they follow the principles of mind power which we discussed in the first chapter of this book. They are part of the thought bricks which form the structures of the mind castle which you wish to build. This means that what you affirm is what you get. The statement that forms your affirmation is your declaration, something which you have endorsed or ratified. This is what it means to *affirm* something.

Affirmation of Action

This has to do with a planned positive action which will result in the achievement of a desired goal. An individual may have difficulty in giving up smoking or in performing other chosen tasks. In such situations the appropriate affirmations which the individual should make would be made as follows.

I will stop smoking now easily, completely and effectively.
I will perform simple physical exercises everyday in order to be fit and healthy.
I will always make determined and resolute plans from now onwards.
I will always finish whatever I start.
The achievement of my goal is guaranteed by my positive actions.

Whenever I make a plan to do something, I see it to the end.
From this moment onwards I will always work hard to maintain my health.
I will give up smoking now in order to regain my strength and stamina!

In the above affirmations, you are making positive statements, you are affirming your determination to finish the work that you have started, stop smoking now, affirming the result of your determination, that is, that you will finish what you have started by seeing things to the end and you are affirming that you will give up smoking now! What happens is that if you have made the affirmation with genuine feelings, the positive nature of the affirmation will stir your mind to positive action which is expressed in your continued positive thoughts and positive attitudes towards your goal to maintain your health or give up smoking whichever is applicable.

With respect to giving up smoking, the result of the combined mental operations is that you will be giving up smoking easily, completely and effectively. Remember the principles of mind power, if you think it and believe it, you will get it because the thought and the belief will provoke you to effective positive action. This is the essence of our powerful statement in the introductory chapter where we said that you will get what you want because what you want is what you get. The emphases is on the verbs, the action words, *want* and *get*.

Affirmation of Thought Bricks

This is mental affirmation. In this affirmation, you use thought bricks with which to construct your mind castles. You make such affirmations mentally to yourself. For example, in our illustration in the last section, *The 60 Cigarettes a Day Smoker* may affirm the statements of plans 1 and 2 constantly and then back up the mental affirmation with positive action to improve his physical strength and appearance. On the other hand the individual may affirm the idea of success and the result of success as follows.

> *I am always in control of my life.*
> *I know what I want and how to get it.*
> *I will get what I am looking for because what I am looking for is what I want.*
> *I will give up smoking because I want to be a non-smoker.*
> *I will stop smoking now because I have a great concern for my health.*
> *I will give up smoking easily, completely, effectively and effortlessly.*

If this affirmation is made constantly it will be retained in the unconscious mind and this will open up new ways for achieving success in the individual's life and ways of achieving the goal to give up smoking easily, completely, effectively and effortlessly.

Written Affirmations

This can take the form of a written out positive plan of what the individual wishes to accomplish in his life. Remember that we mentioned in the last chapter that a goal that is well formulated must be kept constantly in mind. The best way to do this is to affirm the goal constantly. This makes the goal easily amenable to fulfilment.

Take care and affirm confidently and you will be successful in your goal. Remember the five principles which we discussed in chapter one and apply those principles in everything you do from day to day. I expect that from this moment onwards, you will be looking good and feeling good, always.

CHAPTER FOUR
Recapitulation

SOME ESSENTIAL FINAL POINTS
TO REMEMBER

As a follow up to our discussions on affirmations and a fitting conclusion to this book, let us discuss here the essential final points which you must try to remember as these will help you to build your confidence and make you more determined to stop smoking now!

THE LOGIC OF NUMBERS

Always remember that the logic of numbers helps to determine your success in whatever you do. The more times you practise all the exercises in this book the better chance you will have of achieving your objective of giving up smoking. Remember the saying, *practise makes perfect*. You will become perfect in whatever you do the more times you practise on it. Let us illustrate with practical affairs as follows.

Suppose that you are an athlete and you want to improve your personal best (PB) performance on your event. The logic of numbers stipulates that the more times your practise, the better you become in your event. On the other hand, let us suppose that you are looking for a job. The logic of numbers stipulates that if you send out 100 job applications every week your chance of being invited for an interview would be much better than if you send out one job application every week

Remember the saying, *If, at first, you don't succeed, try, try, try again.* This saying implicates the logic of numbers as it is a statement of determined achievers. Perseverance is an application of the logic of numbers. An individual needs to be persistent in what he or she does because it shows a dogged determination to succeed in a chosen objective. The principle of the logic of numbers is a doctrine for determined achievers. The principle is easy to understand and simple to apply in our daily routines. The principle of the logic of numbers is implicated in a general way in the fundamental principles of thought bricks which we discussed in the first part of this book. When you have positive thoughts about your objective of giving up smoking and practise the mental exercises in this book, you will find that you will stop smoking now, easily, completely and effortlessly.

THE MAGIC OF SUCCESS

Always remember that the thought bricks for success in any venture are constructed in the mind. In any situation, if you think you can, you are already on your way to the winning post. It is all in the state of the mind. Your success in anything you do begins in your mind. This is the essence of mind power. The mind is the magic power that a person can use to achieve great success in whatever he or she does. Thus, you must always attune your mind to success and you will be successful in whatever you do. Remember that *the magic of success is truly within you.* It is within your mind. Apply the magic now in your attempt to give up smoking and you will notice that you will stop smoking now easily, completely and effortlessly, almost magically.

THE PITFALLS OF NEGATIVE PROMPTS

Always think positive thoughts about your goals. When you give suggestions to yourself or whenever you make affirmations about your goal of giving up smoking, use positive words that enhance your desire. Always affirm your objectives or whatever you wish to achieve and avoid the temptation to use negative expressions in talking about your goal. Examine the following illustrations.

> *(a) I will not fail to give up smoking.*
> *(b) During tomorrow's meeting I will not be tired and I will not be sleepy.*

You will notice that (a) and (b) above are very negative expressions in terms of what you wish to accomplish. They are about what you will not do and (a) is already talking about failure before the event. In consideration of what you want to achieve the correct, positive, expression should be as follows.

> *(c) I will stop smoking easily, completely, effectively and effortlessly*
> *(d) During tomorrow's meeting I will be wide awake and alert.*

Notice that (c) and (d) above show more determination than (a) and (b). When your suggestions, affirmations or mental prompts are made in an emphatic way as (c) and (d) they become more effective for you. For more discussions on the pitfalls of negative prompts refer to my book, *Mind Castles* (Antony Maurice-Nneke, 2002).

ACTION IS THE ROUTE TO CHANGE

Action is necessary to bring about the changes that you require. If you fail to act then no changes will be made to the existing situation and the lack of change will be due to your lack of action. If you have a genuine, serious, intention of giving up smoking then you owe it to yourself to perform all the necessary actions as advised in this book. Remember the principles of the action plan which we drew out for the *60 Cigarettes a Day Smoker* in chapter two above and draw out a similar plan of action to suit your purpose.

BELIEF IS THE ULTIMATE

Belief is an essential ingredient in a recipe for success in anything you do. You can be a great success in any venture if you believe that you can. Remember that no one is ready for success in any venture until he or she believes that he or she can be successful in it. Remember also that belief is the opposite of doubt. When you have belief you always pursue your goal with a determination to attain the goal. Your belief is a thought brick. You must think constructive thoughts supported by positive actions that affirm your belief. A statement of belief for our purpose is expressed as follows.

- *I have the power to stop smoking now because I know that my success is guaranteed by my belief.*
- *I can get whatever I am looking for because I believe that I can.*
- *I can stop smoking now easily, completely, effectively and effortlessly because I believe that I can.*

When you are able to make such statements as the above in relation to your goals and aspirations, you will know for certain that you are on the way to achieving your objective. We are concerned with genuine belief so the above statements are not meant to be mere verbal utterances. Notice that in the above statements, the action words, that is, the words constituting the actions, such as *stop, get* are all affirmed by the belief.

For our particular purpose of giving up smoking it is important that you have your belief as a mental theory of success. This ensures that when you genuinely believe that you can give up smoking now, your belief guarantees your success in giving up smoking because your belief has been retained in the unconscious mind as a positive and highly effective thought brick. This means that, for you, success in giving up smoking exists as a thought process in your mind and that you are aware of this.

You can see clearly from what we have stated variously here, that when such thought process has taken hold in the unconscious mind, the individual's attitude towards success in giving up smoking, or in any particular venture, betrays the existence of positive thoughts about giving up smoking and about success in general. When you experience such a situation you know that you will always be successful with your goal because your positive attitude towards your goal clearly manifests your confidence and your success is guaranteed by your belief which induces your positive action. Your belief is a spur to an action, it gives momentum to the action which you must take in order to accomplish your goal.

In this way the thought brick which entails your goal is always with you, always in your mind. As you know from our discussions about goals, in order to achieve success with the goal of giving up smoking, the goal must be kept constantly in your mind at all times otherwise you may run the risk of supplanting it with some other wish or desire. Refer to our discussions about goals in chapter two and our discussions about the fundamental principles of our mind technique in chapter one.

Remember that your success in your goal or venture is assured by your positive action to attain the goal. Your coming this far to the end of this book is part of your positive action. Remember that your journey to the world of positive possibilities, at the beginning of this book, helps to set the psychical system in motion to enable you to feel relaxed always. Now put your learning into practise. Repeat the journey whenever it is necessary for you to do so and use the journey to achieve any other goals that you may have. Perform the exercises which are given in this book in order to attain a deeply relaxed mind and body so that you will be always successful in what you do. Congratulations to you for coming to the end of the book. Well done.

References

The references given below are of books which are mentioned in the text

Descartes, Rene. 1641 *Meditations on First Philosophy*
Descartes, Rene. 1637 *Discourse on Method*
Freud, Sigmund. 1916–1917: Introductory Lectures on Psychoanalysis PFL Vol 1
Jung, Carl Gustav. *Collected Works Volume 8*
Maurice-Nneke, Antony. 2003. *The Psychodynamics of The Unconscious.* Intapsy Publications, London
Maurice-Nneke, Antony. 2002. *Mind Castles.* Intapsy Publications. London
Shakespeare, William. *Hamlet*

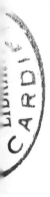

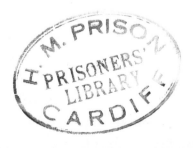

Lightning Source UK Ltd.
Milton Keynes UK
UKOW04f1154090216

268012UK00001B/42/P

9 781609 118372